BUDDHA
BELLY

(A Mind-Body-Soul Approach to Health Starting with Your Gut)

BRITTNEY L. OLIVER CHC

Fulton Books, Inc.
Meadville, PA

Published by Fulton Books 2021

Photo: Meagan Mylan Photography

ISBN 978-1-64952-590-1 (paperback)
ISBN 978-1-63710-000-4 (hardcover)
ISBN 978-1-64952-591-8 (digital)

Printed in the United States of America

To my family for always believing in me, my incredible students and coaches for spreading my purpose farther than I ever could have alone, and my kids for reminding me every day of what a blessing this life is.

Contents

Introduction

Once you make a decision, the universe conspires to make it happen.
—Ralph W. Emerson

EVERY GREAT CHANGE requires a decision. I love Emerson and his life philosophies for a lot of reasons. He was an emotionally intuitive, deep thinker; and I feel that he understood the necessary balance of mind, body, and soul while truly valuing the intangible. I have come to learn that true health is multifaceted and can only be achieved when all aspects—mental, emotional, physical, and spiritual—come into alignment. If we wish to transform our bodies and our lives, we have to nurture all aspects of ourselves.

I am Brittney Oliver, or "Coach Britt" as I am now known, and I started this book originally at the beginning of my health and life coaching career/journey because I wanted to put on paper for the world everything that I had learned from my own healing journey. For the decade prior to becoming a coach, I had considered myself a "health nut," not because I ate perfectly or even ideally, but because I sucked up all the knowledge I could about nutrition, disease, prevention, stress, and anything "healthy" that I could get my hands on! This consisted of hundreds of books and a ton of research alongside my own ever-evolving health choices and health experiences. I've experimented with different foods, diets, and lifestyles as well as observing the health and quality of life in those around me.

A little 411 on my past is that growing up, I was very overweight. I can still remember what it felt like to be made fun of and the feeling of being ashamed through the better part of my childhood. Because of this and my childhood struggles, I developed an emotional attachment to food at an early age that later morphed into a dieting obsession and a constant state of inadequacy. As I got older, I restricted calories and ate minimal amounts of nutrient-poor foods in an effort to lose pounds while counting every calorie burned on cardio equipment.

These naive practices resulted in not only weight loss but also muscle and nutrient loss, and it did nothing for the other demons that plagued me: the severe anxiety and patchy depression that I experienced for as long as I can remember. Although I have never been "skinny," I maintained a healthy weight for most of my adult years. Even into adulthood, I had spent the better part of every day for the majority of my life relentlessly thinking about food and judging my own physical form.

In my early twenties, I got married and focused every moment of free time I had on reading about health and working out. I became a vegetarian. With my dietary shift came improvements in certain areas of my health, but I soon came to understand that my lifestyle was taking another toll on my body. I still struggled with bouts of anxiety and depression, joint pain, and intense sugar cravings. Over that five-year period, I found myself unable to get pregnant; and when I finally did, I miscarried my desired baby. Knowing what I know now, this was a big sign that my hormones were not in alignment, and my stress and attempt to be "healthy" had damaged my adrenals, but I did not give that intuition enough attention. Shortly after my miscarriage, I conceived my first healthy baby boy.

When my son was only one and a half, I went through a painful divorce; and in the few years following my divorce, I remarried and, soon after, experienced another miscarriage. At that point, I started looking into the hormonal implications of the lifestyle I was following and found it to be much less "healthy" than I had thought. A few months after the second miscarriage, life brought a whirlwind of unexpected, debilitating family occurrences at which point my personal health was the last thing on my mind. However, as the Phoenix rises from the ashes, so did I and my family. But I knew that along with the long road of emotional healing, my body needed healing too—and not just physical healing from stress and trauma, but true healing in all areas of my health.

During the unexpected conception of my second healthy boy, my husband and I made the decision to give up my retail business that allowed me to spend time nurturing myself and my family while diving deeper into my newfound understanding of wellness. This decision led me to a new life-fulfilling "career" with passion and clarity. I got my certification in holistic health and life coaching and used it alongside my previous self-education and experience to fuel my knowledge and drive. During this next phase of life, I had come to understand the immense role of the immune system and its origin in the gut, and I learned that our gut health is the key to overcoming so many issues and ailments!

You may wonder why this book is titled "Buddha Belly." It isn't a pun on weight, and honestly, it's not because I am a Buddhist, but because the Buddhist often emulate this multidimensional form of health and have the documented longevity and quality of life to show for it. As a health and life coach, I don't believe in just focusing on the physical body. I have a passion to help people strengthen their physical health while nurturing their minds and listening to their souls. True transformation comes from the inside out, through life-giving foods, self-love, peace, and a personal understanding of who you truly are. This book is to be used right where you are today because now is the moment you've chosen to change your future.

Once a person decides what they desire and gives themselves permission to live it and be it, it will be. I have a healthier mind, body, and soul now, more than any other time in my life, because I gave myself permission to live my intention and made the decision that now it will be so. My passion doesn't come from money or personal gratification, but from an honest desire to empower everyone toward their life's purpose through optimum health, while invoking confidence in each of them to know that they are powerful, strong, and beautiful.

Although it may be a long road toward the outcome, every step along the path will motivate and nurture you to a better place than the step before. Decide what it is you want, make your decision, and may this book be your first step.

CHAPTER 1

What Brings You Here?

LIFE IS ABOUT constantly evolving, meaning that everything is possible. One of my favorite motivational speakers, Anthony Robbins, put it best: "The only impossible journey is the one you never take." Where do you stand today, and what has brought you here? Is it illness, weight problems, anxiety, depression, infertility, struggles with self-esteem, digestive distress, or a combination of these? What is holding you back from living vibrantly in this life? This book's main focus is balancing the gut and empowering the body to achieve its optimal physical state; however, the balancing of life and who we are as people is a crucial component in achieving true transformation.

Is it your desire to improve your physical body, mind-body, or emotional self? Whichever it may be, my wish is for you to see a healthy evolution in all of these areas by the end of this process. There are many "diets" out there, but the intent behind this book is aimed at achieving a healthy state of being, using the most crucial tool to physical health, the GUT, while nurturing your mind and body into the best version of itself. Diet-related issues are rarely just a lack of knowledge about what to eat. The psychology behind eating behaviors is quite complex, and through my personal experience, it requires a different approach.

When I was halfway through my certification as a holistic health and life coach, I had the pleasure of meeting an interesting woman who had written many diet books. After engaging with her about her accomplishments, I then told her about the direction I was headed with my program. After asking about the specific course that I was taking, her first response was "health *and* life coaching? What an odd combination. I've never heard of that before." My program was the only one that offered both a health and life coaching certification, but I found her remark enlightening. Bless her heart, here was a woman with years of experience in holistic health and writing who had some excellent dietary knowledge yet appeared to have little understanding of what I call the "mind and soul" part of health. Because of the interconnection between life and health, I couldn't personally understand why these two areas of coaching hadn't been married earlier!

To understand health from a natural, holistic perspective, it is important to understand that the body is an intricately designed machine. To function well, it must achieve synchronicity with not only its physical self but also its mental, emotional, and spiritual self. This is why it is crucial to listen to the body's communication. Symptoms such as insomnia, fatigue, depression, anxiety, infertility, excess weight, irregular elimination, skin problems, food allergies, and headaches are all examples of the body sending you signals that something more complex is out of whack. Unfortunately, in our modern age, we are taught to seek medication to "Band-Aid" the signal, instead of following it to the source. Think of these bodily cues like a smoke alarm. What good would it do for us to just remove the batteries every time the smoke alarm went off? Sure, it would stifle that high-pitch annoyance, meanwhile allowing a fire to potentially consume our home and loved ones—not worth it. Your body works just like the fire alarm, alerting you of danger before it's too late. I personally don't believe any symptoms or suffering happens without a deeper root cause, which is worthy of investigation.

The great thing about our magnificent bodies is that they are resilient and want to heal. Even some of the most far-gone bodies are in a constant state of repair. What we need to do is let the body do its job by nourishing it properly, nurturing it, and loving it through the process. As overwhelming as the journey may feel, especially if you are suffering from multiple symptoms and conditions, we must keep in mind that what's important is that you start somewhere. The understanding and theories about where many of these symptoms originate from are evolving by the day, especially within the holistic community.

So many people seek out diet programs and workout regimens—some healthy and some not so much—in order to heal or change their bodies to no avail. Being hungry and stressed out is no way to live, and neither is counting calories. Seeing yourself critically with negative judgments and poor self-esteem is no quality of life either. Many Americans live on what I consider "prescription life support," meaning they function "fine enough" but are dependent on daily pharmaceuticals to keep them alive. This prescription hamster wheel comes at a cost with not only negative side effects but also the consequence of a further damaged gut lining and liver.

With the evolving knowledge we now have about the human microbiome, or "gut," we are able to understand that by balancing this area of the body, we have the potential to improve or heal the entirety of symptoms in the majority of suffering individuals. So much damage has been done to the human gut with processed foods, chemicals, and an all too accepted level of chronic stress. It's time to educate our society about the importance of a healthy microbiome and the severe issues brought forth by a modern lifestyle so that we can find hope in our bodies and our future. We deserve to live with less reliance on prescription drugs, and we need to stop wasting moments watching life pass us by without being a thriving contribution to it. This life deserves to be lived, and we deserve to learn how to love ourselves throughout the process.

Whether you picked up this book looking to lose weight, emotional distress, and digestive distress or to see simply out of curiosity, thank you for joining the growing number of individuals who are empowering the rest of the world to jump on board and educate themselves, refusing to accept a mediocre or poor quality of life, and living in fear of cancer and disease. Listen to your body when it speaks. This will be important to remember throughout this process because it will enable you to decipher the current state of YOUR body and use the information to navigate the best approaches for YOU.

CHAPTER 2

Is Your Gut Making You Stronger or Weaker?

IT'S NOT NEW to hear about how disease is on the rise in industrialized cultures. Type 2 diabetes continues to be one of the top ten killers and unfortunately is now affecting younger and younger generations. Fifteen years ago, finding a child or adolescent with type 2 diabetes was rare, and now it's become so prominent that they changed the name from "adult-onset diabetes" to "type 2 diabetes." It is not a coincidence that this, along with heart disease and cancer, has risen consistently with expanding waistlines, processed foods, and modern lifestyle.

We don't live in the same world as our grandparents did. The average child's diet in the United States consists of approximately seventy-percent processed food. This means that majority of what our children and many adults are consuming isn't even real food! It's "food-like substances" colored in pink and blue and marketed in a box as "breakfast." It's sugar-loaded drinks and frozen hunks of additives and poor-quality animal protein shaped like dinosaurs. The saying "everything in moderation" has been an unfortunate disservice to our culture. Moderate amounts of substances that don't even classify as food are different from occasional amounts of real butter, fat, and unprocessed sugars. The "everything in moderation" rule is now providing a quick ticket to a damaged inner ecosystem, especially because the average person believes many artificial foods to be within the "healthy" category. While most people understand the correlation between poor diet, inactivity, and modern disease, a new understanding of how these negative behaviors impact our microbiome and thus influence our susceptibility to disease is an emerging discovery. I personally give credit to the underground wellness community, the group of holistic practitioners, naturalists, and the like who have made a mission of questioning the root causes of these conditions and how to prevent and heal them, instead of just "Band-Aiding" the symptom.

The role that the gut plays in disease is incredible, and despite this wealth of knowledge, there is still so much more to learn. First is a quick explanation of the human microbiome "gut." The body's microbiome is a partner to the genome (genes). The human microbiome is a combination of live microbial bacteria and outnumbers the number of genes from ten to one. Yes, we are more bacteria than we are human genes! The intestinal tract and entire gut consist of multiple types of bacteria—some good and some "bad." The ideal ratio of good bacteria to bad is eighty-five percent good to fifteen percent bad. This allows the immune-strengthening bacteria to have the upper hand against disease and sickness. Not surprisingly than that, the average individual eating the standard American diet has a bacterial balance of fifteen percent good to eighty-five percent bad. This ratio sheds a lot of light on the epidemic levels of rising illness in industrialized cultures. Our good bacteria represent our "fighters." These bacteria are the ones we want to fight off all the scary stuff. If the average person is walking around with a pitiful representation of an immune system and is already overwhelmed with the "bad guys," then how are we supposed to take on foreign invaders like the flu, not to mention a larger, more debilitating illness? Now, when I refer to the "bad" bacteria, I don't mean that they are all actually bad. In small, controlled amounts, many bacteria that we consider problematic are actually a necessary part of our microbial balance. For instance, there are a few strains of *E. coli* bacteria, some of which play an important role in producing vitamin K within the intestinal tract. These bacteria are critical to maintaining balance within the gut and, in return, the entire body. All bacteria have a role, and when the "good" bacteria are present in the right quantity and ratios for an individual, they will naturally keep the other bacteria and foreign invaders in check.

People who get sick a lot most likely have an off-kilter microbiome. What causes poor microbial ratios? Many things do, one of which is antibiotics. The word antibiotic literally means "against life" and is used for the purpose of killing bacteria. Unfortunately, antibiotics aren't discriminatory and tend to decimate everything in their path, including our "fighter bacteria" who are generally the most delicate. Don't get me wrong—as natural as I am, the discovery of antibiotics has saved countless lives and is a blessing in our modern world. With that said, I personally don't let them near myself or my children unless it's absolutely necessary or other natural methods have not worked. In the nine years of my oldest son's life, he's been on antibiotics once for an ear infection as a compromise with my ex-husband, one that I still regret being bullied into. My five-year-old, on the other hand, hasn't ever taken any. I didn't eat healthily while pregnant, birthed unmedicated, and breastfed for nothing! Those hard-earned microbes are precious, and as a mother, I am conscious about wiping them away with antibiotics, especially for what is often a viral infection, where antibiotics are useless anyway. This is why self-education is so important, especially for parents. The human body was designed to do incredible things. For this reason, educate yourself and be discriminatory as to what you allow in the bodies of you and yours.

Food or "food"

Another microbial destroyer is obviously a modern diet of processed, highly chemical-laden "food." Although processed foods existed throughout the twentieth century, it wasn't until the 1950s that they started consuming the American household (no pun intended). The influx of fast-food restaurants and highly processed frozen cuisine provided easy meals for the average busy parent, and with the depression era over, families could afford these modern meals instead of relying heavily on plant-based garden foods like beans, rice, and veggies. Products were advertised as "fortified" meaning they contained synthetic vitamins, which manipulated the public into believing that these foods could qualify as a healthy addition to their children's diets. Many well-meaning parents and even working women who were new to the workforce at the time embraced this propaganda believing that these foods were merely a convenient way to nourish their families and alleviate their burden of cooking.

A while back, while digging through some old pictures and keepsakes, my mother came across a written recommendation from her childhood pediatrician, advising my grandmother to start adding Jell-O to my infant mother's diet. Aside from the benefits of gelatin that you can obtain from much healthier sources, there is absolutely no reason to feed an infant or any child, for that matter, processed, sugar-laden, artificially colored, and full-of-preservatives Jell-O! The consequences far outweigh the benefits. Yet this was "sound advice" from a trusted medical professional, and because of this, many well-intentioned parents followed suit without further research. In fact, still to this day, nutrition is hardly addressed in the medical setting, and nutrition education isn't even a required part of medical training for most doctors in the United States.

"Real, healthy food doesn't come with a food label." The additives and ingredients in processed foods have a detrimental effect on the human gut. In a previous article by Dr. Mercola, he talked about the difference between the types of sugar consumed and inflammation, which is present in chronic diseases such as diabetes, heart disease, and stroke. Simple sugars increase inflammation markers in the blood, whereas the nonstarchy, complex carbohydrate sugars found in fruits, vegetables, and whole foods actually reduce these markers.

Not only do processed foods contain additives and unhealthy types of sugars, but also they are often full of unhealthy fats such as hydrogenated oils. These oils are basically a vegetable oil injected with hydrogen molecules, allowing it to sit solid at room temperature. This same process also allows it to sit solid in the walls of our arteries, further exacerbating a chronic state of inflammation. With so much junk floating around in convenience foods and causing destruction to our beloved microbiome, we must keep in mind the importance of choosing more foods that don't have labels.

Our modern lifestyle is playing a major part in worsening gut health. The high stress, constant "go, go, go" mentality, and financial pressures have caused a massive cortisol imbalance contributing to leaky gut, which is why I have devoted an entire chapter in this book to stress and its relationship with gut health. Along with the use of antibacterial soaps, chemical cleaners and body care, pasteurized animal products, pesticide-laden foods, and pharmaceuticals, the human gut is losing the war against disease—the war it was created to fight for us and our well-being. Those antibacterial soaps do just what they promise: to kill bacteria, all bacteria, including the good. Pasteurization of raw milk has stripped the probiotic benefits out of dairy, rendering it void of most of its originally beneficial nutrients. Pasteurization has mutilated the enzymes leaving it with very little health benefits, especially considering the antibiotics and hormones now presently used in current dairy production operations.

The massive negative implications of nonorganic foods, processed and sprayed with chemical pesticides, are something that can no longer be ignored. Nonorganic foods are treated with insecticides and pesticides designed to keep infestation off of crops and bugs away from our food. Unfortunately, anything designed to kill a bug will wipe out our positive bacteria and has no place in our food. Genetically modified foods are often bread with insecticide now in their DNA! Between nonorganic foods along with hybridized, genetically modified foods, the tomato of yesterday hardly resembles the tomato of today, and your body knows the difference.

We are killing our microbiome with painkillers and pharmaceuticals

Painkillers and pharmaceuticals have become all too easily prescribed and obtained. Sometimes, it is necessary to take a painkiller, but we've gotten too used to relying on them for every ache and pain. Those headaches, muscle aches, and pains are usually the body communicating to us. Not only are we using a pill to "shut off the alarm," but also we are causing more depletion of our bacterial reserves. Studies have shown that just two weeks on an NSAID (painkiller) has a seventy-five percent chance of causing intestinal permeability or leaky gut. In addition to contributing to leaky gut, painkillers are hard on the liver. Your liver is your body's filtration system. Your gut and your liver go hand in hand and both need to be functioning smoothly for optimal health to occur. For healthier options, herbal tinctures and holistic remedies have been around for years and have proven quite effective in pain management while being a less destructive option for your liver and your gut.

We get it from our mama!

We get our first solid dose of bacteria when passing through the birth canal of our mothers. Her bacterial flora is the first inoculation we are introduced to which starts the process of building the immune system. Needless to say, if the mom is lacking in this area, the baby will likely get subpar bacteria. When birthed via C-section, the baby will miss this initial process almost entirely. Dr. David Williams enlightened his readers with the stats of declining microbial bacteria in proceeding generations, basically showing that our poor diets have led to a poor bacterial gut balance that we are passing on to our children, who pass on even less to their children, and so on. All the while, chronic disease keeps climbing. For those who know the importance of exposure to maternal bacterial flora, many are choosing to "seed" their babies after C-section. This process involves swabbing the newborn's ears, mouth, and body with bacteria from the mother's birth canal or vagina. I think this is an amazingly intelligent idea, and with luck, this practice will hopefully find its way into mainstream medicine.

Starting here

This book is a massive step toward improving your immune system, and through the process, don't be surprised if you experience the shedding of pounds as well as a multitude of other symptoms including anxiety, depression, and mental health. The gut is now being referred to as "the second brain." Michael Gershon, the author of *The Second Brain* and chairman of the Department of Anatomy and Cell Biology at New York-Presbyterian Hospital/Columbia University Medical Center, is an expert in the nascent field of neuro-gastroenterology. He explains that the second brain has a multitude of neurons that enable us to "feel" our insides. These neurons allow the intestines to act separately from the brain such as the involuntary contracting involved in digesting and moving waste and food. It is also responsible for the majority of the serotonin produced in the body.

When the body is nourished and the gut is functioning well, it will be obvious in multiple aspects of a person, from physical improvement to mental and emotional health. Hopefully, you now have enough understanding of the human microbiome to appreciate all the emerging information surrounding it and feel motivated to strengthen your own inner ecosystem. The reason so many individuals improve their diet and lifestyle but still don't see the level of improvement they are striving for may be that they haven't healed the root of the problem: the quality of the gut. It's time to embrace "germs" in the right way and use them to protect ourselves from illness and disease so we can get to fully living.

CHAPTER 3

Leaky Gut

WHAT IS "LEAKY gut"? Leaky gut is a term used to describe intestinal hyperpermeability and the range of issues associated with it. When the gut lining becomes permeable, it basically becomes filled with holes much larger and out of control than nature intended. A healthy digestive lining is like a fine netting, letting chosen nutrients through and into the body while keeping foreign substances inside the digestive tract where they can be eliminated properly. When this "net" is damaged, the holes become larger, thus allowing objects into the bloodstream that the body wasn't made to take on. The presence of these substances in the blood firstly overtaxes the liver, causing it to filter substances that should have been filtered in the gut. Because the liver can't possibly keep up with this level of filtration, the floating debris now awakens the body's immune system to prepare for a full-blown "attack."

This attack is very hard on the immune system. When intestinal permeability is left untreated, only to further worsen, the body's constant state of fight leads to chronic inflammation. Inflammation occurs when the body sends white blood cells into its tissues, inflaming them in order to protect itself from damage done by foreign substances. This is a protective action; however, if constant debris such as food particles are entering the blood a leaky gut, constant inflammation will occur. Think of this as having a fever every day of your life. Inflammation is an immune response and has been found to be present in most if not all chronic diseases such as diabetes, cancer, heart disease, depression, and digestive-related issues like IBS. With the presence of inflammation consistent with so many chronic diseases, healing a leaky gut not only has the power to reduce inflammation but also prevent or reverse these epidemic levels of disease.

"Leaky gut" has been a controversial topic between holistic practitioners and the typical medical community:

> "Leaky gut syndrome is a hypothetical, medically unrecognized condition which some alternative health practitioners claim is the cause of a wide range of serious chronic diseases, including diabetes, lupus, and multiple sclerosis. Proponents claim that poor diet, parasites, infection, or medications cause damage to the intestinal wall or lining, permitting toxins, microbes, undigested food, or other substances to leak through. According to the hypothesis, this "leakage" prompts the body to initiate an immune reaction that, in turn, leads to chronic diseases such as those mentioned.
>
> —[1]

> The "leaky gut" hypothesis is vague and largely unproven, and the scientific community continues to debate whether "leaky gut syndrome" exists at all. There is no credible evidence that any chronic diseases are caused by a "leaky" gut, nor that any remedies marketed for its treatment bring the benefits they claim.
>
> —*Wikipedia*

> "Leaky gut syndrome" is said to have symptoms including bloating, gas, cramps, food sensitivities, and aches and pains. But it's something of a medical mystery. "From an MD's standpoint, it's a very gray area," says gastroenterologist Donald

Kirby, MD, director of the Center for Human Nutrition at the Cleveland Clinic. "Physicians don't know enough about the gut, which is our biggest immune system organ."

"Leaky gut syndrome" isn't a diagnosis taught in medical school. Instead, "leaky gut really means you've got a diagnosis that still needs to be made," Kirby says. "You hope that your doctor is a good-enough Sherlock Holmes, but sometimes it is very hard to make a diagnosis."

—Web MD

As you can see, the topic is touchy for some. It often appears to be a "Which came first, the chicken or the egg?" situation. Is leaky gut really elusive and unspecific, distracting us from an acute issue? Or is leaky gut a very real side effect of poor diet and lifestyle, which sets into motion all following disease?

Many highly respected and highly educated medical doctors support the ladder and fully believe the leaky gut "theory." Dr. Josh Axe has done immense work on this topic, after watching his mother's cancer return shortly after her conventional medical treatments of chemo and radiation. As a physician himself, Dr. Axe talks about taking time off to spend with his mother upon the return of her cancer, to "do something more natural." He then had her follow a strict gut-healing plan, and her oncologist was shocked to watch her tumor shrink consistently until she no longer had a mass. As of the writing of this book, she currently lives vibrantly free of cancer.

Sometimes, it takes disease in ourselves or those close to us to find the motivation to dig deeper and find the root of our suffering, especially for those already indoctrinated in the current medicinal practices. In his book *Clean Gut,* Dr. Alejandro Junger describes his own physical issues with illness, weight, and blood pressure. What was very interesting however was his emotional account of his own severe depression. He saw that conventional treatment using pharmaceuticals were not "curing" the problem, but "Band-Aiding" the symptoms, leading to more issues and a further need for pills and potions. He then went on a spiritual as well as physical "detox" over in India. While there, he meditated daily and followed a strict gut-healing diet. After leaving the facility, he was 15 lb. lighter, and his depression had lifted along with his dependency on prescriptions.

Despite modern medicine's skepticism, the many people like Junger who have transformed their bodies and their lives through healing their gut are enough to give it merit. As Dr. Junger points out, some individuals have deeper-lying issues such as parasites or heavy metals that will stand in the way of a full recovery; but through the process of gut healing and the assistance of functional medicine, these things can be discovered.

I am not a medical doctor myself and always recommend that my clients work with a doctor (functional medicine doctor preferably) if they are suffering from severe symptoms so that deeper issues can be addressed and avoided and the right combination of supplements and medications can be administered safely. Even then, most people should still be able to follow a gut-balancing protocol without conflict.

Leaky gut is a result of living against what nature intended

What causes leaky gut? Sometimes, it feels like the shorter explanation is, what doesn't? An abundance of real organically produced fruits and veggies and moderate amounts of wild (or as close to wild as possible) animal products along with quality sleep will NOT give you a leaky gut! Long walks in the woods, breathing fresh air, and daily quiet meditation or yoga won't give it to you either. These examples are the balance nature intended for us: to be swift but not rushed, fed for nourishment but not gluttony, and surrounded by companionship with gratitude for the daily gift of life.

As discussed in Chapter 2, we have come a long way from this primitive yet simple way of life. A constant deadline, rush-hour traffic, and an overbooked schedule have left our cortisol levels (stress hormones) skyrocketing. The lack of time for quality in our relationships as well as our food has left us undernourished and disconnected. Because we have come so far from healthy balance, the thought of healing ourselves can feel overwhelming, but the key is to start somewhere. So, let's start with food.

The food we eat has had major consequences on our gut

Gluten (a protein found in wheat) is a big offender. Gluten is hard to digest for a lot of people and absolutely atrocious for others. The word gluten actually comes from the Latin word "glue." For people with gluten sensitivity, eating gluten causes the immune system to go into hyperdrive and actually destroy the gut lining leading to leaky gut. People with celiac disease, which is an allergy to gluten, experience horrific side effects such as vomiting, weight loss, and, eventually, if left untreated, death.

Even those without celiac disease, however, are still largely affected by the substance. Today, many forms of gluten-containing foods such as wheat, barley, and rye are hybridized, meaning the genetic makeup is altered from its natural state. This is done to achieve pest control, climate tolerance, and profitability. Dr. Amy Meyers states that it is estimated that five percent of the proteins found in hybridized wheat were never present in original wheat at all. What is the result of consuming this "new" wheat? A form of nutrient that the body is already sensitive to now becomes unrecognizable. The immune system will now call an attack at some level. Mankind currently overconsumes gluten in the form of processed foods. Other "Frankenutrients" and the constant immune response to our foods and the foreign contaminants are tearing our guts apart.

Corn, for instance, is a highly gut-irritating food, especially because ninety percent of corn is genetically modified and used for high-fructose corn syrup (HFCS), a chemically processed, concentrated form of sugar made from genetically modified organisms (GMO) corn. This "sugar" syrup has now taken place of most typical sugar in processed foods and is present in everything from cereals to ketchup and bread. The response to HFCS by the body is not the same as authentic sugar. The body is intelligent and knows this substance is a foreign chemical; therefore, like with gluten, it reacts differently. High-fructose corn syrup does not trigger the same satiation response in the brain (the cue that you've had enough). This is especially concerning because almost all soda is produced using HFCS.

In my opinion, one of the fastest ways to shut down your pancreas and become a type 2 diabetic is to drink sodas and sugar drinks. Not only is it full of "chemicalized sugar," but also drinking it throws it into your system with absolutely no fiber to slow it down. I'm not a perfectionist, but as a mom and health educator, I strongly preach against letting your children drink sugar unless you want to give them a fast track to a hospital bed, wreck their gut, and ensure their early dependency on pharmaceuticals.

The fake stuff is no better

Artificial sweeteners such as saccharin, aspartame, and sucralose are a chemical, not a food. Many countries don't even let these ingredients across their borders because of the potential health consequences. These sweeteners are found in all diet sodas and "sugar-free" processed foods and should be absolutely avoided. Not only can they trick the body into producing the insulin it doesn't need, but also they easily cause sweet cravings from other sources as an attempt to stabilize low blood sugars. Along with their counterintuitive effects, they are also very dangerous. Studies have shown links between artificial sweeteners and odd tumor masses on the brain and side effects such as vision problems, seizures, MS, and cancers, and that's the short list. Rather than take up an entire chapter discussing the pitfalls of artificial sweeteners, I will encourage you to seek out all the information you can, if this is an area of concern for you. The documentary *Sweet Misery* is highly informative and will make you think twice before that next sugar-free, latte. Just remember "sugar-free" means "chemical-rich."

Our food is loaded with chemicals

Chemicals and preservatives used to extend the shelf life of packaged foods are another offender causing a similar attack by the immune system. Natural, healthy foods not only are label-less but also rot. In order to give foods excessive shelf life, packaged foods are made with preservatives. Although natural preservation methods exist such as canning and smoking, most packaged goods are preserved by using chemical substances to keep the food "shelf-stable." This is why some forms of "food" look identical to the day they were manufactured after a ridiculous amount of time has passed. Having chemicals like these roaming the walls of your arteries not only is toxic but also stresses the body like a slow embalming process. Certain baked goods that shall remain nameless have been documented to hold their shape and texture for years! Trust me, your gut is worth more than a fluffy, cream-filled, chemical concoction.

Another word about pills

The usage of pharmaceuticals has absolutely wreaked havoc on the microbiome. Common painkillers such as aspirin, ibuprofen, and naproxen wear down the protective mucosal lining of the gut. This not only leaves the guts precious "netting" more exposed and vulnerable to damage but also irritates the gut bacteria, throwing it off-balance. As addressed in Chapter 2, the presence of positive gut bacteria is of utmost importance. When we weaken these pro-lifers, we allow an overgrowth of parthenogenic bacteria. Gut microbes also respond to pharmaceuticals differently. A study in the *Pharmaceutical Journal* explained that gut microbes react to painkillers and prescriptions in a multitude of ways such as producing toxic by-products, activating or inactivating drugs by altering how the drugs are metabolized by human cells. According to Ramy Aziz, a microbiologist in the faculty of Pharmacy at Cairo University, "You can give two people the same drug, and they will respond differently. And it's not because of their genes but because of the difference in the microbes they carry."

Signs of leaky gut

Signs of leaky gut can be few or many. Because bacterial quality and quantity differ from person to person, along with the extent of permeability, symptoms can vary both in manifestation and severity.

A few examples include chronic digestive problems (gas, bloating, and irregular elimination), nutritional deficiencies, poor immune system (getting sick frequently), headaches, excessive fatigue, skin issues (rashes, eczema, or acne), sugar and carb cravings, arthritis/joint pain, depression and associated mental challenges (attention deficit hyperactivity disorder), and autoimmune diseases (rheumatoid arthritis, lupus, celiac disease, and Crohn's disease), just to name a few.

When the body starts attacking itself

Autoimmune diseases are particularly frightening and on a steady incline. Autoimmune disease occurs when your immune system, which is meant to fight foreign invaders, mistakes your own healthy tissues as foreign and calls an attack. This will happen in different areas of the body depending on the type of autoimmunity. For instance, a thyroid disorder is when the immune system attacks the thyroid, and rheumatoid arthritis is where the immune system attacks the lining of joints and sometimes even the eyes, skin, lungs, heart, and blood vessels. As listed previously, there are many forms of autoimmune disease; however, the question that still begs to be answered is, Why are they increasing? You may be surprised to know that autoimmune disease affects 24 million Americans. So far, eighty diseases have been classified as autoimmune, and the list keeps growing. Collectively, this becomes a scary reality, especially because some of these include things like MS or muscular sclerosis where the immune system eats away at the protective covering surrounding the nerves, leading to painful bouts of debilitation and possibly taking years off one's life. In conventional medical treatments, we have been taught that more medication is needed to treat the symptoms of these diseases, without guidance on how to decipher and treat the root cause.

Dr. Mark Hyman is one of many who has been very outspoken about his position on functional medicine (a form of medical practice focusing on the root cause and working therapeutically with the patient to address the true issue). He has spoken about what he believes is needed to heal most autoimmune disorders, even the ones deemed by the medical community as "incurable." He has his patients follow a list of dietary and lifestyle changes, including treating leaky gut and searching for underlining issues such as parasites and heavy metals. He even lists adequate sleep as an important factor in a healthy healing process.

Although the cause of autoimmunity is still claimed to be unknown, we can assert that like many "western diseases," it has risen with our industrialized ways of life such as food, lifestyle, environment, and stress. So why would it seem so impossible that perhaps we can do something about it? We not only can prevent it from occurring but also can lessen or completely reverse the suffering of currently diagnosed individuals. There is at least enough momentum now from the holistic community, giving us plenty of information and allowing us to make our own educated opinions about how our care will be handled and what it can look like in the long term.

Mental illness isn't just in your head

A lesser acknowledged symptom of leaky gut is mental illness. The prevalence of depression and anxiety in western cultures is heartbreaking. For those who have seen the consequences of this affliction, it can be a traumatic experience. Rather than be oneself or a close friend or loved one, these types of diseases hurt and sometimes take lives. Ninety percent of serotonin (the happy hormone) is made in the gut, yet every day, more and more people are prescribed gut-damaging antidepressants and antianxiety medications, only to continue suffering. Now that we've discovered the brain-gut connection, hope in winning the battle over mental illness is a very real truth.

Because of the prevalence of leaky gut and all that is believed to be associated with it, *Buddha Belly* focuses on this area of the physical body while connecting it to mind/body health. My personal passion is helping others recognize these connections while discovering balance and love for their own bodies.

What to expect

At the end of this book, you will be provided a six-week protocol, a recommended food list as well as tools for hacking your own gut! But before you get to that part, there are some basic things to prepare for. Although you will be eliminating many foods and "foods" from your diet temporarily or full-time, first, let's focus on what you'll be adding in.

Veggies, especially high-nutrient, organic greens, need to be a huge focus at your main meals. I like to fill about half my plate with these types of veggies, not only to give me amazing fiber and energy but also to fill my belly with bulk. You should never starve your body. It's important to remember this when making significant life changes.

Morning smoothies start your day off right. When you get into the habit of blending these up first thing each day, you'll be nurturing your body and your mind without even thinking about it. This has a substantial effect on how the rest of your day will go! I have provided a couple of my favorite smoothy recipes in this book but feel free to experiment. Remember you need a healthy base (nut milk, water, or coconut water), healthy fat (coconut oil, chia seeds, or avocado), optional fruit, optional protein, and TONS of greens. Starting with these two tips will make this process smoother for you and start you off with an excellent amount of nutrition designed by nature.

Other key components of balancing your gut will be *removing allergenic and toxic foods*, adding *healthy probiotic sources*, discriminate use of *supplements, healthy self-perception, stress control,* and *adequate sleep.* Instead of focusing on what you are removing, focus on what you are creating. You have chosen to create a healthy, vibrant body and mind. And because you have made that decision, all that's left is to nurture the body accordingly while it does its job.

CHAPTER 4

Food Sensitivities and Allergens

There is a wide range of allergies and intolerances

WHEN IT COMES down to it, an individual could be sensitive to a number of things in their foods, environment, home, animals, etc. This is why an "elimination and focus" regimen like the one outlined in Chapter 11 is so critical. It allows you to pull common allergens and toxic substances from your consumption as well as your environment so that you may restore your gut and your well-being. Doing this while staying "in tune" with your body will allow you to strengthen your gut lining while also making you aware of the things that it really doesn't like.

After balancing your gut, you may be able to tolerate some of the previously removed foods at different degrees, so keeping a journal throughout this process will make navigating those foods much easier. The most common allergenic whole foods are dairy, wheat/gluten, and peanuts. Eggs are also common irritants, but we have allowed farm-fresh varieties during this period. If you think you have an issue with eggs, then please choose not to consume them while you follow this plan.

Other irritants include soy, legumes, and corn. Due to their high glycemic load (how fast a food turns to sugar) and potential for aflatoxins, we have asked you to remove all grains. Quinoa is the one exception to the rule, due to its high fiber content, low allergy profile, and lower glycemic load. It is technically a seed. We exclude legumes from the initial portion of this process because beans and legumes contain phytic acid, which, although fine in moderation, can bind to the nutrients in the food making them much less nutritionally beneficial. I do encourage the trial of properly prepared beans and legumes during the reintroduction period. Testing how the body responds to different legumes may reveal a new tolerance to their occasional consumption.

Once the four weeks is through, you will start a reintroduction approach, where you will experiment with one whole food every four days and see how your body responds. This is when it will be especially helpful to journal throughout the day about your body and mood. Your body will react in different ways to different foods, so knowing what to look for will be essential.

How are so many people allergic to "healthy" foods?

Humans weren't made to be so intolerant to whole foods. Allergies have become so predominant in our culture, largely due to a few things, one being leaky gut. When the gut is overly permeable, food particles make their way into the bloodstream, an area of the body they would not have otherwise seen. So even common foods like eggs or whole unprocessed wheat can now cause major inflammation by running awry outside the GI tract. The human body was originally designed to retain food particles within the digestive tract only. This allowed the absorption of nutrients and then elimination. With so many people suffering from leaky gut nowadays, negative reactions to everyday foods are a common result. Because of this, however, once the gut is healed, some foods may become tolerable once again.

Another cause of food intolerance is genetic modification. GMOs are the result of spliced DNA. Basically, the genes of a plant or animal are combined with the genes of an unrelated species such as bacteria, viruses, insects, animals, or even human genes. This process results in what I have called "Frankenfoods" or "foods" that never existed in nature. The goal of this splicing is to achieve effects that were difficult or unobtainable in the natural plant or animal such as withstanding the application of herbicides. Many GMOs even produce their own insecticide.

Genetically modified organisms are banned in the majority of developed nations. So why then does the United States insist they are safe? It's most likely due to the "trials" showing they are safe for human consumption. Ironically and not surprisingly, these trials are done mainly by the corporations creating the product in the first place. That's like asking my children to monitor and control their sugar intake in a free-for-all candy store!

Even most livestock that were originally meant to consume grass and bugs are fed GMO corn and soy products. This adds to the amount of GMOs and pesticides that the average person consumes when they are also found in their meat, milk, and eggs. In the documentary *King Corn*, one farmer explains that on a diet of corn, a cow will not live past six months. Because cattle were not meant to consume corn and soy, it will take only six months for this diet to kill them. Since they are slaughtered before that, the industry pays no regard to this fact, and Americans keep consuming sickly animal protein.

GMOs have only been around for a short while. They entered our food supply in 1994 in the form of the "Flavr Savr tomato." Since then, GMOs can now be found in most processed foods. The time span of which these foods have been in the American diet has not been long enough to truly know the long-term implications of their consumption. The current premillennial generation has basically become the test subjects of chemical, scientifically produced "food." Even in this short duration, we still have enough information to connect food sensitivities to GMOs. Many people with an intolerance to say soy may be able to tolerate an organic, non-GMO variety. With what we know about the body's immune system, we can be certain that feeding ourselves these unknown, unnatural substances is a surefire way to rev up an attack on our gut.

A "gut attack" or intolerance may be subtle or quite obvious. An initial reaction may be immediate or take a day to show up. It may be simple like excess gas and bloating or severe such as migraine or odd skin rash. Oftentimes, you will feel when you are intolerant to a certain food. You may get sluggish or lethargic after a specific meal or irritable. You may burp or hiccup a lot, which is a sign of impaired digestion just as is acid reflux. One obvious sign is your elimination patterns. Do you get diarrhea after a certain food or backed up for a few days? These are all examples of potential food reactivity or at least a reaction to the way the food was grown or created.

Although you may find yourself able to tolerate a few foods again after the elimination period, you may choose to keep some out indefinitely. Knowledge is power, and once you know the line that our modern food system has crossed, it may be hard to consciously impact your body so negatively. Keeping your food organic and as close to home as possible is an excellent way to stand against GMOs and processed foods as well as supporting your local farmer, local economy, and physical health in the process.

Gluten and dairy are some of the highest on the list of food intolerance and growing allergies. They have been altered a lot from their original raw and nonmanipulated form, and the body isn't being fooled. Many people who are conscious of their microbiome will choose to steer clear of both gluten and dairy indefinitely, but you will have to choose for yourself.

The most important piece of understanding intolerance is the ability to listen to your own body and what it is communicating to you. Your body will tell you when it needs help, when it doesn't like something, and when it does. Don't ignore it. Bodily communication is an intricate mechanism that was given to us as a gift of protection. Pain happens for a reason. If you touch a hot surface, you get burned, and you will feel pain. Your body just told you to avoid touching hot things in an attempt to protect you. Headaches, joint pains, digestion issues, skin problems, anxiety, depression, and sleep issues are all happening to protect you. They are letting you know that something isn't okay before it's too late. Your body wants to be healthy! It wants to repair and thrive, and it knows how to do it; it just needs you to listen.

CHAPTER 5

Think It in Your Mind, Feel It in Your Gut

HAVE YOU EVER heard a song or driven by a certain place that brought back a strong memory? Whether it was good or bad, can you remember how you felt or where you felt it, literally? Where in your body do you feel your emotions? From time to time, life gives us a little nudge into the past—a message from the subconscious. When this happens, we somewhat "relive" that moment emotionally and physically. It's the reason why we hold on to that mix disc from our summer in San Diego, which when listened to brings back nostalgia, or why we can't stand the smell of a fragrance worn by someone associated with a negative memory. The body feels our thoughts and sometimes stores emotions deep within our subconscious.

Researchers in Finland conducted a study of 700 participants and asked them to focus on 14 different emotions. The study required them to color in a chart of the body, showing where they felt activity and where they felt the absence of it. The results varied a bit from person to person but still showed similarities. I find this study compelling not because of the similarities but because of how easy it seemed to be for all those people to connect those emotions to their physical body. I recommend trying this yourself. Imagine a time when you've felt extreme joy, sorrow, or fear. Take a minute to go back to that moment and what it really felt like. Where were you? What was the weather like? Was there music playing or a show on TV? Now, notate where in your body you feel the energy from that feeling. It is highly likely that you will pinpoint a physical sensation or a few of them in specific places on your body. These places are where we feel different emotions or energy. It's actually scientific, believe it or not. Just like how they can read different colors within the brain matter, our bodies are made of energy and heat, and it can be seen visually as well as felt. Doing exercises like this will help you become aware of the physical responses to the things you feel while strengthening your mind/body connection.

The mind/body connection is no joke. The only reason we feel pain is because the brain receives information from the inflicted area of the body via nerve fibers and thus interprets that as pain. On the reverse, when we see someone yawn, we often yawn ourselves, calling this a "contagious" reaction. This is why the term "mind-body connection" is used so frequently, especially in the holistic community. Understanding your mind-body connection is crucial to balancing your gut.

Ninety percent of the body's serotonin is produced in the gut. With mental illness climbing at rapid rates, this knowledge is very important. The subject of mental illness hits home for me as I myself had suffered from anxiety and depression for years. I have also watched many loved ones and friends be consumed with these horrible afflictions, only to blame themselves and shut themselves off from the world. Not only the person with the illness, more often than not, but also the ones around them are suffering. A child with a depressed parent does not get the best of their loved one and can often pay in long term for the experiences endured during their childhood.

Children with depressed parents often show signs of depression themselves but more often show defiant behavior such as acting out at school or home, appetite problems, anxiety, and sleep issues and are more apt to have chronic depression in their teens and into adulthood. As sad as this is, most parents would never wish their ill-health to affect their children. It is just an unfortunate side effect of a situation that already feels hopeless. This is why the gut-brain connection is so huge! It gives hope. Along with counseling and physical activity, healing the gut has the power to heal what pharmaceutical antidepressants have only masked. The gut has intense power over the well-being of the mind, and the mind has power over the gut, which is why *Buddha Belly* focuses on a healthy mind-body approach to balancing both.

Of all the science that exists around the concept of mind-body, I feel it is important to speak freely and REAL regarding this topic. All the scientific explanations in the world won't make you more intuitive or self-aware. To really tap into your mind-body, you need to be able to quiet your mind and your surroundings enough to hear what your body is communicating to you.

Your body speaks to you constantly—time to start listening

As we previously discussed, listening to the body's physical communication regarding the effects of foods and substances and listening to the emotional cues it sends you are equally important. Depending on the person, this awareness may come easily or be rather difficult.

Having an intuitive, deep thinking personality, I never understood how self-awareness could be so foreign to some. Then I experienced my first real, professional counseling session. My counselor did an amazing job of dissecting my emotions and behaviors leading me to many new understandings of myself and my root feelings. Through this process, I was humbled into the realization that although I am very deep and self-analytical, there were parts of myself that I had not understood or even identified—areas where I "shot in the dark," so to speak, about my emotions and where they resonated from. I had tied certain feelings or behaviors to specific "reasons" and thus hadn't dug deeper. Through quality, professional therapy and my own openness, I now see life much differently.

It's hard to come to a realization such as I did, and not change. A little humility goes a long way. You may not feel that you have anywhere to budge, but I feel that true personal evolution occurs once you're able to acknowledge that you will be forever evolving. Resisting humble self-awareness will only stunt the growth of your soul, thus holding you back from life.

Your inner voice

Your soul has a lot to tell you, and it uses your emotions to do so. Emotional reactivity is like a string tied to a phantom object. That object is a box that holds something essential to the soul's growth. For instance, the woman who holds a disdain for a woman who happens to be more educated than herself, regardless of how friendly that woman is, could benefit greatly from identifying the true reason behind that emotion. If she chose to acknowledge her negative thoughts toward the other woman, she might ask herself exactly what it really is that she is feeling. And why does she feel this way? The answer may be surprising to this woman. Maybe she feels insecure when around someone she perceives to be "smarter" than herself. Maybe this insecurity comes from a personal regret or being berated in this area by someone she cared about like a parent or loved one.

Once we make these connections, we grow. We become aware of our weaknesses and our scars instead of hiding or ignoring them only to let them smolder and perpetuate our insecurity. This acknowledgment leads us to healing. Although healing our emotional wounds benefits those we come in contact with by eliminating the unconscious lashing out, it especially benefits us. Negative feelings and thoughts come from a place of hurt. Your body wants to thrive in ALL areas including your soul. Negativity is a venom that first poisons our insides and then carries on to poison those within our reach. When you heal the holes in your heart, you will live happier and healthier.

True health is mental, emotional, spiritual, and physical. While it's critical to tackle the food part, it is just as important to focus on your mind-body health by cleaning up your thoughts. Since emotions are relative, meaning they are what you make them, you can control a majority of the energy that is dispersed throughout your body or at least the extent of its effect. Along your wellness journey, you will be faced with many emotions: body image, self-confidence, faith, determination, fear, etc. Learning how to handle these moments will empower you through your personal transformation.

Your mind can affect the way you see life

Become VERY aware of your thoughts and feelings. What goes through your head when you think about your accomplishments, identity, body, and challenges? What do you think/feel when you are around a variety of people similar to or different from yourself? If journaling helps you with this process, then please write it down. Each day, if you have to, reflect on the day and journal all your thoughts and emotions in any given situation.

The truth will set you free! Be honest with yourself. The only way to heal the root of your pains and emotions is by being candid about where they are buried and the signals they are sending out. I hate to break it to you, but we all have our own skeletons and our own kind of "crazy." I believe that the people who judge others the most actually have the most digging to do within themselves. So, have no shame. You are becoming a better, healthier person as we speak and let me be the first to tell you from the bottom of my heart I AM PROUD OF YOU!

I have two exercises or techniques that I routinely give people who are struggling with common worry, self-esteem issues, or negative thoughts in general. The first is the 2-lb. rule, and the second is the "I AM" ritual.

The 2-lb. rule is when I coach someone to become aware of their thoughts and emotions in three categories: positive, negative, and neutral. Positive thoughts consist of happy thoughts, optimistic feelings, or uplifting thoughts and feelings about others or yourself. Negative thoughts are those that put down or criticize others or oneself, view situations pessimistically (glass is half empty), and anything that has a generally negative tone. Neutral feelings and thoughts are observational such as "The sky is blue" or "That person is sad." Neutral thoughts have no intention, positive or negative, and don't invoke much of an emotional response.

Now I must state that I strongly dislike our society's constant obsession with weight. I find the focus on the scale to be misleading when practicing strength training activities (muscle weighs more than fat), taunting while trying to focus on patience through your transformation, and berating to one's self-worth in general. However, because most people I work with are desiring improvement in this area, especially women, this technique works well.

Imagine that each thought you have, of yourself and others, will affect your weight on a scale. For every negative thought, you will weigh 2 lb. more than you did before that thought; and adversely, for every positive thought, you will lose 2 lb. physical weight. For neutral thoughts, your weight stays the same. Take a moment to really receive this idea. Envision your body being an obvious indicator of your thoughts and judgments, especially toward yourself. Next, implement it in your daily life. Practice using this technique next time you look in the mirror or find yourself in a social situation. Not only will this provoke your self-awareness, but also it will invoke an increase in positive thoughts and behaviors while helping bring more peace and less judgment into your daily living.

The "I AM" card is another affirmation and identification-based strategy. Once you start focusing on your true emotional roots and their origins, you will be able to name many of your greatest fears and insecurities. The reason this is so crucial is that once you discover the negativity in your thought patterns, you can start to reverse it. The subconscious mind controls so much of our lives and truly believes everything it's told. If you tell yourself you are stupid or ugly, the subconscious holds on to that like a sponge, transforming how you see and feel about yourself into exactly what you have articulated. Letting fears constantly roam your mind will have a similar effect also, causing you to behave in a way that can end up manifesting those fears.

I like to use the example of the person with a strong attachment to a fancy car. How many times have you seen that individual nervous about door dings or damage park at the far end of a parking area, only to have someone clip their bumper while every other vehicle was left unscathed? This goes hand in hand with the law of attraction. What you put out, you will receive. Projecting positive thoughts and handling fears in a healthy fashion will allow less of the things you fear into your life.

To start, fake it till you make it!

Speak what you desire the outcome to be and against your fears. Using the "I AM" card is an easy way to implement this strategy. Firstly, write down your top five biggest fears and insecurities on one side of a two-column piece of paper. For example, "I am insecure about my body," "I am afraid of being alone," and "I am not good enough at my job." Then, in the other column, write down the opposite of the first column; for instance, opposite to "I am insecure about my body" is "I am confident with my body and feel healthier every day." Once you have filled out the reverse column, print only the positive affirmations on a small card. Keep this card easily accessible in a safe place like a wallet. Pull it out and recite these affirmations daily—multiple times a day if you need to. Whenever you feel overwhelmed by one of these burdening fears or unhealthy thoughts, just use the card. Your head will catch up to what it is you speak and in return will heal your heart.

CHAPTER 6

Stress Is Killing You

You should sit in meditation for twenty
minutes each day, unless you are too
busy; then, you should sit for an hour.

—Old Zen proverb

THE AVERAGE PERSON knows that stress isn't healthy. I find that most people I talk to agree that stress is just as much of a culprit behind disease as poor diet. However, knowing and doing are two separate things. It's always easier to put off until tomorrow what should be done today until tomorrow never comes and the damage becomes extensive.

Stress comes in multiple forms, but scientists have categorized it into three different types: acute, episodic, and chronic. Acute stress is a short duration of stress and can be positive or negative. Being very excited about a presentation for work or "jazzed" about a business idea or vacation is acute stress, as is being nervous about that same presentation or flight and just wanting it to be over with. This type of stress tends to only last momentarily. Acute stress can cause a range of symptoms from anxiety and irritability to stomach issues and more.

Episodic stress is similar to acute stress but in a frequent form. An individual who makes the same stressful commitments on a reoccurring basis might experience episodic stress. Unlike chronic stress, episodic stress ceases from time to time but remains a frequent occurrence. "Type A" personalities are a great example of this type of stress because a constant need for organization, control, and sense of competition causes them to create their own reoccurring stress. Symptoms of this type of stress range from a constantly worried and highly agitated, manic state of being to long bouts of depression.

Lastly, we have chronic stress. Chronic stress is by far the most damaging of them all and mainly consists of negative stress from unhealthy situations. Abusive relationships, unfulfilling careers, and a toxic home environment will create a state of chronic stress. Chronic stress happens when miserable life circumstances seem unrelenting and hopeless. The effects of chronic stress are almost endless. Some common signs are headaches, stomach aches, pounding heart, anxiety, and depression—the list goes on. Although all forms of stress need to be monitored, chronic stress poses the most damage to our bodies, our well-being, and especially our gut.

Life, in general, plays a part in all areas of the stress we experience. Some contributions are in our control, while others have been bestowed upon us, with or without our consent. Take childhood for instance. When an infant enters this world, they are like a sponge, and despite a parent's best efforts, that sponge will absorb everything it comes in contact with, forming who and what that infant grows into as an adult. Nobody's childhood was perfect, but some have been dealt a shorter stick than others in this area. The effects of chronic, unrelenting stress are deadly to the healthiest of adult bodies. Imagine what this type of stress can do to a vulnerable child.

In his book *When the body says no*, Dr. Gabor Mate catalogs his time spent working with patients on end-of-life care. He draws specific ties between severe disease and stress, mainly in the form of chronic stress. He interviews many of his patients about their life experiences and their emotional coping styles. Many of his patients could be classified as chronic stress sufferers—people who were unable to draw healthy boundaries for themselves or who were subjected to traumatic childhoods consumed by fear and lacking a sense of control. A heavy number of the patients referenced in his book are those dying of cancer or other severe diseases such as ALS. Many of them are astonishingly young. He does an excellent job of making you think. Hearing about a twenty-two-year-old woman with small children, dying of cancer, is enough to wrench your heart and stop anyone in their tracks. Childhood trauma isn't addressed much when it comes to physical health. Mental health will reference and take into consideration the environment in which a child was raised, but physical health often won't. It is really important that we seek counseling or some form of therapy for past trauma so that we can let the entire body realign. We can't change the past, but we deserve the opportunity to heal ourselves so that we can experience a healthier future.

Evaluating your stress

Who we are today is a culmination of a whole life's worth of experiences. Just as it is important to pay attention to our emotions and thoughts, we must also acknowledge our stress as well. Doing so will allow you to differentiate between unhealthy coping mechanisms (responses to stress) and truly unhealthy aspects of your life. Basically, is it your job that is stressing you out, or is it you who is creating the stress that will ultimately follow you wherever you go? When we pay attention to this part of living, we become much more present and able to navigate healthier habits for our daily lives. Doing so not only causes you to feel more peaceful but also brings a calm state to the body, aiding in a healthier functioning physical self.

If you need an example of this, just look at our presidents. The age progression throughout their time in office is a testimony to what I can only assume is stress-related, accelerated aging. Most likely, it's brought on by the lack of sleep, poor quality of nourishment, and excessive stress. It has been debated as to whether or not stress can cause the hair to turn gray; however, I think that the examples speak for themselves.

A little science about stress

The science behind stress is compelling. When our body experiences the feeling of stress, it goes to work. The hypothalamus receives the body's threat signal and relays that to the nervous system, which gets the heart pumping, lungs breathing, and the stomach going. Stress literally affects your gut immediately, as well as in long term. While in a state of stress, digestion is among many things hindered so that all the energy can go toward adrenaline or the "fight." Blood is actually detoured away from the gut in order to maximize the muscles and "fight" reflex. This is why a chronic state of stress leads to a deteriorated microbiome, one that has had restricted blood flow and therefore function. A whole host of functions slows way down to allow the body to produce the immediate physical response necessary to escape perceived dangers. You can probably see why a frequent or constant state of stress can absolutely age and hinder the body. It's not being allowed to perform its functions fully for long periods, and on top of that, it is being overtaxed with adrenaline and cortisol.

Cortisol is a word that most people probably associate with belly fat. We hear it mentioned in commercials selling diet pills and articles about stress in our favorite magazines. It is actually a hormone produced by the body in response to stress. But did you know that cortisol has also been linked to memory malfunction, bone density problems, blood pressure, weight, and more? It has shown a strong tie to depression and lower life expectancy. A recent study even showed a link between elevated cortisol and mental illness, especially in adolescence. Cortisol builds in the blood for the purpose of "fight or flight," but without the normal sequence that nature intended, such as running from an animal, cortisol just builds in the blood causing damage to the whole body. We are experiencing the destruction of our own bodies due to the very survival mechanism that was designed to save our lives, and for the most part, we only have ourselves to blame.

A lack of balance in the areas of work, play, health, personal time, creative time, and relationships has become the "norm." Sundays used to be a day of rest, and home-cooked family dinners around the table were a staple of many households. Now, grabbing fast food to eat in the car while off to another scheduled commitment has taken the place of what used to be valuable quality time. Time to engage with your family over a nourishing meal provided not only connection but also consistency. This change has been the unfortunate outcome of traded time. Time is a highly valuable thing in this life, along with health and love, all of which don't come with a price tag. That's not exactly true though. We trade time for money every day—hours of our life in exchange for monetary wealth.

Living to work

As of March 2016, the average work per week per person in the United States is 34.4 hours on the clock. It sounds normal, right? Except that average is just that the average of all workers, both part-time workers such as students and overworked adults. In addition, the average commute time is 3.75 hours per week, which puts us at an average of 38.15 hours per week working and commuting. Remember this is the average, which means most Americans are working much more than this! Then, add in all the fun home chores—laundry, cooking, cleaning, and grocery shopping—all of which we will estimate at about 3 hours per day for 21 hours per week. Of the 168 hours in a week of our life, the average person donates 60 hours per week to just work and chores.

That leaves 108 hours left for sleep and life as we wish to make it. Since our bodies truly benefit from 8–10 hours of sleep a night (let's say 8), after work, chores, and much-needed rest, the average person is left with 52 hours per week or 7.43 hours per day. I like to call this time "living time" because that's the hours you have for things outside of obligations and responsibilities. In the United States, of those hours, an average of 4.56 hours is spent watching television or on media. This leaves us with 2.87 hours per day. No wonder we're stressed and depressed! The average person has under three hours per day to get outside, perform physical activity, spend quality time with friends or loved ones, or have any quiet time with their thoughts. Time, love, and health—remember? One might question if this is actually even living. For those who work more than the average, their "living time" is even less, and they likely lack adequate sleep. You only have one life, and only one body to live it in.

What's it all worth anyway?

It is commonly stated that the American household cannot live on a single income. I'm not debating whether or not this is true for some, but I do feel that this perspective is highly subjective. Aside from those working minimum-wage jobs, personal choices continue to dictate how much we "need" to work. Just as you added up your lifetime, (the time you spend working, cleaning, etc.), you also need to add up how much of your work time is paying for needs versus just funding excess. Our basic needs include food, water, shelter, heat, and clothing. Outside of these five basic necessities, there are then practical "needs" such as a vehicle to commute to a job that may be a significant distance away or medical insurance. These things aren't necessities for survival, but they are justifiable expenses. With that said, holding down a hefty car payment for a fancy new vehicle versus paying cash for a basic car that runs efficiently is where justifiable turns into excessive. Now don't get me wrong; there's nothing wrong with where one chooses to spend their money, and no one has the right to judge another. However, this is where we start adding up the cost of time.

Say you get paid for the 34.4 average hours worked per week and you make $12 per hour. This equates to $412.80 per week, minus 15% taxes, leaving you with $350.88 per week, or $10.20 per hour. Let's say that the payment for that new car is $350 per month, or $87.50 per week. Divide that by your hourly income, and you will see that you work 8.6 hours per week just to pay for that car. The average person's workday is 6.88 hours per day, so technically, you work about 1.25 of the five days just to pay for that car.

The purpose of laying out all the numbers this way is to help put into perspective what we trade our time for so that we can make conscious decisions regarding the disbursement of it. Remember back to the 7.43 hours that the average American has per day? Take away that car payment by purchasing a used vehicle, and you now added 1.23 hours to your "living time" equaling 8.66 hours per week. Start adding up credit card debt and the mortgage for a home that is more than what is needed for your family size, and you'd have a heck of a lot more time! Maybe you could afford to work a job that is more enjoyable to you for less pay because you have minimized your expenses. We have choices. While one person may live minimally so that daycare for their children isn't needed, another may be comfortable working more in order to afford the vacation home that they enjoy with their family during their downtime. Conscious evaluation will allow you to make choices that you can be comfortable with and identify the areas of imbalance so that you can work toward putting them in alignment.

Finding a little joy in simplicity

I believe the soul resides in simplicity. That's why we feel at peace when in nature. When we live simply, we are free to thrive in more *living* and less work. The more stuff you have, the more you need to work to maintain it, and the more time you must dedicate to cleaning and maintaining it. A good rule of thumb is "time or money?" Rarely are both an option. At the same time, each individual or family may have a different idea of what is enough and what is worth working for. For one person, a boat and all the expenses that come with it may be a ridiculous thing to trade time for especially depending on the average weather in their location. For another person, that same boat may be how they spend the majority of their free time, and that provides a source of quality time with their family. They may sacrifice in many other less common areas in order to have this. The concept of "enough" is something that can only be navigated by you. This is your life, your time, and your memories.

For me, personally, I hate cleaning, especially dishes, but I need a clean house. My idea of "clean" has evolved since having children, but I still have a hard time being peaceful in a cluttered or dirty home. My solution to these conflicting issues is to own a minimal amount of stuff. I have yet to achieve the level of minimalism that looks so amazing on all of my Pinterest boards, but it continues to evolve. I feel as though I am forever purging something. I have a fairly simple, versatile wardrobe, kitchen utensils and appliances that

I absolutely use, and few cluttered possessions. My preference is "I'd rather do than have," meaning I'd prefer to get outside for a hike or even go out to dinner with a friend than buy stuff most of the time. Figuring out how to simplify in the areas that contribute to your stress will repay you handsomely in either more peace, time, or money—possibly all of them.

We could learn a lot from the distant world!

Thankfully we are a species of comparison, and when the world around us is out of sync, we seek examples of a better way, even if to just take notes. This can be hard to find in an industrialized, fast-paced, "live to work" society. Fortunately for us, there are many groups of people around the world who have not "evolved" much from their ancestral roots. In John Robbins's book "Healthy at 100," he documents his travels around the world to a few different groups of people—generally, cultures living in isolation. Robbins documents the high amounts of centenarians among these people and details some of their daily life through his experiences while staying with them. He not only ties a lot of their health to diet but also touches on their lifestyle and community.

Many of these people work until they die, but not in the way we would assume. The goat herder, for example, swiftly climbs the steep mountain well into his nineties, on a consistent basis, so that his goats may graze. The terrain is intense, but his body is acclimated, and his spirit is high. He enjoys the outdoors and doesn't possess the same job-related stresses we associate with "work." He's diligent, but not rushed. And in a world like this, there is no such thing as "higher productivity." Most typical jobs are designed for productivity. The more you do in less time means more money, and when one goal is met, another is quickly set. Constantly focusing on achieving MORE is draining on the body and makes simple work-related tasks much more stressful.

In small cultures, such as the ones referenced, the people often "work" for their food and well-being, not monetary compensation, and are often accompanied by friends, family, or community all doing the same thing. Imagine if your job consisted of tending your garden and other necessary home needs while your spouse and children pitched in and then you break to share meals together. Even though these are long days, the ambiance of these environments sounds much more peaceful and life-giving than an American nine-to-five. Happiness was noted as being a contributing factor to the longevity of life in these regions as well as a highly alkaline diet and community.

In a world full of technology, towers, and heavy machinery, our bodies still crave simplicity to some degree. This is why when we envision a sandy beach or a small cabin in the woods, we feel a sense of calm. Noise and the constant bombarding of ads and media while navigating five o'clock traffic is enough to send your nervous system into overdrive and your cortisol levels through the roof.

Taking more "downtime" where possible can help undo some of the damage modern living has inflicted. I often sit with no TV on and read a book while sipping tea or do yoga in my designated chill space while listening to my favorite music. In these moments, I feel peaceful and content, and nothing feels healthier than peace. When in a peaceful or neutral state, the body and mind have a chance to rest and rejuvenate. Making time for these life-giving moments will benefit not only your gut but also your entire health.

And then we meditate

Meditation is an incredible way to nurture your body and alleviate stress. Meditation is defined as "contemplation, thought, reflection, or prayer." Taking quiet time to meditate has considerable effects on your health. In a Harvard study, meditation was shown to actually alter the brain by preserving it from aging, improving focus, reducing overall stress, encouraging creative thoughts, and rivaling pharmaceutical effects on anxiety and depression. It is astounding to see the number of studies done on such a conceptual practice. I have found science to loosely acknowledge things that don't swim in front of a microscope. These studies however do measure brain activity and behavior changes that are visible-proof.

Meditation is a practice that has been around for centuries. Traditional meditation is usually associated with the Buddhist monks who were the first well-documented practitioners of meditation, but some researchers speculate that it goes back to hunter-gatherers who may have discovered this altered state while staring into the fire. It would be silly to mark a spiritual practice like this with a date of creation because it is a personal practice and experience that may look different for everyone. Although meditation is a strong part of the Buddhist faith, the very definition of meditation includes focused thinking and prayer in general. No matter what your personal belief system, you can find a place for meditation because it is a focused quieting of the mind or conscious control over thought. Take time to still the mind or direct your thoughts in a healing way, such as gratitude, affirmations, or a good heart-to-heart with God. It is a nurturing moment. If you could hook up to a machine while doing this that would measure your heart rate, blood pressure, and brain activity, you would see firsthand that the body needs this time and rejuvenates when given the opportunity.

If you are new to the concept of meditation, don't be intimidated. There is no "right" way, and the more you practice, the more natural it will become and actually addictive! The addiction factor comes from experiencing how good it feels to be peaceful and alive. You will eventually learn to use this as a tool to combat a hard day or rough patch in life or even to just indulge yourself because it just so happens to be the healthiest way to do so.

Meditation isn't a place; it's a mental and spiritual experience and therefore can be done anywhere. However, I recommend making a cozy place in a corner of your home or wherever you have space. A yoga mat or even a pillow is nice to sit on. You can use essential oils to help you relax, such as lavender, or play peaceful music or nature sounds as well. Try to make your meditation space simple and clean so that there are fewer distractions. Even if you have to face a corner and forget about the mess behind you, that will at least allow you to focus on the moment without the dishes intervening in your Zen.

Next, sit comfortably—relaxed and with a straight posture. Practice breathing deeply and slowly while quieting any mental chatter. Focusing on your breath will help distract you from a busy mind. Once you have calmed your mind, the rest is up to you. Maybe this is a chance to pray. Maybe you use this time to envision a sandy beach and ocean waves in order to entice the body into a peaceful state. Positive affirmations are a great addition as well. Start with five-minute sessions and work your way up to what you feel is needed on each individual day.

If you are anything like me (a little "type a"), you may find it difficult to make time for meditation, which probably means you are especially in need of it. During my coursework, one of my assignments was a month-long self-nurturing practice of specialized eating and daily meditation. I had a far easier time with the restricted diet than I did with the daily meditation. As much as I wanted to, making time for me was incredibly difficult. I often forgot or was so caught up taking care of the family that it didn't happen. All the while, my body craved more self-nurturing.

Months later, I made a decision. I had let my life get way too off-balance. My husband's work priorities and the needs of my three kids had taken the majority of my time, and although blessed, I was getting irritable and in need of a little peace. That's when I decided to start my month of meditation. I made a time each day during which the baby would sleep, where I would meditate. What this month taught me was priceless. I couldn't alter the circumstances or my priorities at the time; in fact, five minutes each day was sometimes all that I got to myself. But I could make that time count. I referenced this experience in the chapter "Testimonials" because for me, the experience affected my state of well-being just as much as my eating habits had. Loving yourself enough to nurture your body from the inside out will alleviate the burden that stress has inflicted and allow positive growth to occur naturally.

CHAPTER 7

Loving Yourself and Nurturing Your Body

You can't nurture something you despise

LOVING YOU AND appreciating your body is so important on a true health journey, especially while awaiting results. I like people to think of their physical bodies like they do their children. Could you imagine telling your child that their little baby rolls are "gross" or looking at your teen dressed up pretty for prom and saying, "If only you could lose another ten pounds, maybe you wouldn't see those love handles"? Or how about men: would you say to your growing son, "You won't be good enough until you look like that guy"? Absolutely not! The negative repercussions of their self-esteem and confidence would be insurmountable! Yet, we talk to ourselves like this every day. Every time we stand in the mirror and criticize what we see or put ourselves down in public or alone, we are berating our inner self. This behavior teaches your subconscious to believe the negativity and ultimately manifest it, resulting in depression, stress, and low self-esteem and eventually costing you your physical health.

No amount of makeup, perfect clothing, muscles, or weight loss will ever give you true confidence or self-esteem. This can only come from a deep appreciation and understanding of yourself and a desire to nurture your body out of love. Loving yourself and your body doesn't mean that you have to be happy with everything about it. It means you love yourself at the soul level and understand that the physical part is just a result of the level of nurturing you've done. Your physical body should be used as a tool for measuring how well you have loved yourself thus far. View extra weight as a symptom because it is. Your weight has nothing to do with who you are— nothing about your body does.

It is important to distance your emotions with regard to awareness of your physical attributes. They are all markers of your life, both good and bad. Extra body weight often indicates challenges with diet and lifestyle, yes, but deeper issues such as self-medicating emotional wounds and stress are also to blame. In order to heal this area, we need to heal the root cause that is contributing to the symptom of excess weight, and you can't get to the root if you are busy feeling self-conscious about the symptom. At the same time, the nose that you dislike was passed on by many others before you—relatives who had an impact, even if indirectly, on your journey. Embrace your unique traits by affirming their beauty for what they stand for. Your traits tell your story. Accept the weight on your body as part of your life up to this point and have peace with it knowing that at this moment, you are evolving and changing for the better.

Some physical changes such as those left from childbirth can be significant, but they are a reminder that you carried life within your body. I find this area to be the biggest struggle for most women I talk to. Pregnancy sometimes leaves changes in the skin as well as the weight that, despite one's best efforts, may never be what it was prebaby. As frustrating as this may feel, trust that by nurturing your body with life-giving foods, healthy activity, a positive environment, and positive thoughts, your body will align itself right where it needs to be, at a healthy weight for you, with strength, energy, and happiness. Doesn't that sound amazing? Feeling content in your skin is only part of it. Once you let go of a self-perceived "ideal" image, you can relax and actually enjoy your healthy body, because a healthy mind will accompany it; and often, you will look healthier to the world around you as well.

If only we could all view wellness in the same light. One of the most disheartening things about being a health coach in this current world is the subliminal messages that perpetuate self-hate. In a world more concerned about perfect abs than cancer prevention or self-esteem, it makes pioneering true health that much more diffi-cult. I define *true health* as a balanced state of well-being, mentally and emotionally as well as physically. Mentally you should feel neu-tral and peaceful a majority of the time, with an ability to focus when necessary, and most of your thoughts should be of a positive nature. Emotionally, you should feel even keeled and be capable of express-ing yourself healthily while also knowing when to seek professional help in areas that feel consistently hard to tackle.

Even a healthy person won't handle life's situations like this all of the time, but a balanced, aware person will possess these character traits more often than not, as well as a desire for further self-growth. Perfection will never be achieved in anything, so don't let that inter-fere with your positive stride. Some days, I look at my life and how I think and act, and I see how truly far I have come. Other days (usu-ally a rough day when I wasn't my best), I feel as though I'm right back where I started. This isn't true though. In those moments when you feel as though you have backpedaled, it is more often a sign that you are more aware of your state of being now and you desire to be better than you have been before. That is progression.

Lastly, the most obvious benefit is the aspect of physical health. When your physical body is healthy, you should experience level energy throughout your day, quality sleep, rare sickness, good skin, healthy digestion and elimination, and of course a healthy weight that is optimal for your body. Now this is where it gets tricky. Many people, especially women, chase the weight part of health when, in reality, weight is just one of many symptoms of health. By solely focusing on this one aspect, you are neglecting all of the other areas of health. Far too often, a quest for a physical number or body image leads people to partake in things that are actually quite harmful to their true health and their gut. Restricting calories, overexercising, using diet supplements, and even surgery are often used to create an ideal physique. These practices rob you of true health and usually lead to compulsive behaviors, making a state of peace unobtainable.

No one person is the same; however, everybody needs nurturing. You need to eat, move, and rest. Failing to treat your body right will result in a decreased state of overall health and usually fail to deliver the superficial results desired in the first place. Overexercising can be a form of self-abuse and is considered a disorder under certain circumstances. There was a point in my life where I can remember spending two hours on a piece of exercise equipment in an attempt to burn every calorie I'd eaten that day. Not only was that irrational and unhealthy, but also it slowed my metabolism by decreasing my muscle mass, causing my body to hold onto fat much easier thereafter.

Throw away your scale

Focusing on weight as a marker of health is as silly as paying thousands of dollars for a car with a pretty paint job without checking the engine. It's impractical, and yet we live in a society that encourages this misguided preoccupation. Why? Because "wellness" companies make a lot of money off of our insecurities and naivety in regard to actual health! The amount of money spent annually on diet programs and products is huge, and yet the health of the nation is on a consistent decline. I believe this is mainly due to two reasons: One is that people want a quick fix, which causes them to seek diet products with simple promises while degrading their long-term health in the process. Secondly, the average person is uneducated about what true health actually looks and feels like, so they easily get caught up in what media and manufacturers paint it to be.

Don't be offended by this. Large food operations and product manufacturers go to extensive lengths to mislead the public's understanding of what is safe and healthy. Navigating through the garbage could be a full-time job. I personally feel that no one should ever take a diet or appetite pill. Aside from being potentially very dangerous, most are ineffective. No pill or product will teach you how to eat and live in a nurturing way, nor will they give you the tools to a lifetime of true health. True health is only possible when you make the choice to love and focus on all aspects of yourself, not just your weight.

What does your best body look like?

At the age of thirty-one, it finally clicked for me. It literally took that many years for me to figure out that instead of telling my body what it should look like and trying to manipulate it to fit that ideal, I needed to sit back and focus on nurturing my body in all areas and let it tell me what ideal looked like for me. Odd concept, isn't it? The need for control can be so counterintuitive for our well-being. Sometimes giving up control allows for acceptance to transcend into peace. This becomes possible when we direct our actions toward nurturing health. By providing your body, without restriction, everything it needs to thrive, it easily will. Now it is up to you to appreciate the outcome. Don't get me wrong—if you want to do some focused strength training so that your biceps look nice or your booty fills out your jeans better, be my guest, but no physical goal should come at the price of your health. Ignoring the body's need for rest or nourishment in the name of a leaner you isn't true health. Comparing yourself to others or sacrificing balance will only send you backward from how far you have come.

Everyone has a different body type, and if each person focused first on balancing their gut health as well and their true health, the outcome would still look different for everyone. Some people will gain muscle or lose fat easily, while others may struggle a little more. Just because the best you may not look like what you've been striving for up until now, it is a beautiful body that now comes with a healthy state of being. With that said, you might be surprised at just what the final product of YOU actually looks and feels like—the best—that you might outdo your previous expectations. Enjoy the visible improvements while you continue to progress in other areas.

You should notice clearer skin and healthier hair and nails. One of the most encouraging improvements at the beginning of balancing your gut is the lack of bloat, caused by improved digestion. This may come at different times for different people. Some individuals will experience bloating until their bodies become accustomed to the increase in beneficial bacteria from the probiotics, as well as increase in fiber consumption. During the initial phase, you will likely experience some form of "detox" symptoms. When your body detoxes from things such as sugar, it can be a rough experience. Symptoms like lethargy, runny nose, odd cravings, and irritability are common but will clear up once your body kicks out the junk. These discomforts are no reason to refeed yourself these substances. The withdrawal symptoms are your body's way of cleansing itself from foreign chemicals and toxins. Soon enough, you should feel "cleaner" and more energetic. At that point, the road gets smoother, and it is much harder to put junk into your body once you experience how amazing healthy feels.

Pack the magazines away with the scale

Focusing on superficial images can be discouraging. I personally find "fitspiration" (sites and pictures of men and women in competition shape) to actually do quite the opposite of motivation. I feel that for most people, these sites and blogs cause people to judge themselves even harder and distract them from focusing on their true health. I don't judge what someone enjoys focusing on or showing off, but I understand the immense role of the subconscious and its effects on behavior and self-esteem. More often than not, images such as these evoke inadequacy rather than motivation, causing a myriad of negative self-talk, which, as I've mentioned, will hold you back on this journey. I will also add that I have trained myself, and while I didn't get into competition shape, it was awesome seeing what some strategic, disciplined weight training did for my body and my mind. At that time, I could appreciate those bodies without feeling defeat about my own, but that was because of where I was mentally and the growth I had made personally in my self-perception. For most individuals, I'd advise you to put away any kind of advertisements, media (including social media), and anything that tempts you to be critical of yourself. Criticism won't get you anywhere but frustrated and depressed. The future best version of yourself needs to be uplifted and encouraged in order to blossom. A flower can't bloom in the dark, so in order to keep your mind right, avoid or limit anything superficial that doesn't give life to your true health. Rather than focusing on images of six-pack abs and perfect thighs, instead, set physical goals in the form of achievements, such as perfecting your yoga practice or improving your lifting technique. By directing your attention toward new exciting goals and activities and a supportive community, you'll strive for improvements in a positive light, and your body's strength and physical form will follow suit.

Positive-focus fitness and health is what I call this type of non-dieting, and it is honestly the easiest way to lose weight and improve body image. I consider the typical kind of "dieting" ("If I eat less and squat more, maybe I will like my body") negative-focus dieting and fitness. It is easy to tell the difference between the two because one makes you feel great no matter where you currently stand and the other bullies you into exercise and eating as a form of self-abuse. This type of negativity tells you that you aren't good enough and only when you achieve (insert self-criticism here) will you be able to be happy. No wonder making positive strides with our health and weight can seem like an impossible dream! Apologize to yourself for all the times you've let this negative focus dieting treat your body and your mind like garbage and embrace a new way toward health through self-nurturing and positivity.

I believe most people, especially women, practice negative focus dieting and health. The interesting part about this is that it affects people of all shapes, sizes, and ages. Regardless of the current state of a person's form, diet, or body fat percentage, their health could be severely lacking. When I get a group of participants together for gut health groups, I love seeing a variety of people. Unlike most weight loss programs, I have men and women at all stages of life and with a variety of body types. After the program gets going, I love to see people relax with each other, realizing that they are all there for the same reason no matter how different they may feel from one another. Each person is there to achieve their own true health. Each individual has recognized that something about their way of living is robbing them of experiencing true well-being. The person who you feel so inferior to may be struggling with severe insecurity and self-destructive behaviors or miserable digestive distress. Now I am not a psychologist, and I openly discuss the benefits of a good counselor when dealing with deep-rooted issues, but I do play a big role in helping people self-analyze. Doing so is a major component in gut and life balancing.

Wear it as though you love it, and don't forget to smile

There is nothing more attractive than real confidence—the kind you see in people who just look comfortable wherever they go and however they look that day and the person who easily says hello with a smile and isn't intimidated by the environment around them. We are easily drawn to this kind of person for their energy, and that energy is attractive because it's a quality most people wish to have. There is, however, a fine line between confident and conceited. Someone who is conceited may appear to be confident, but in reality, this confidence is a show to cover up unresolved self-esteem issues. Someone who acts this way will usually spend a lot of time talking highly of themselves in an unconscious attempt to get you to see them in a certain light. If this person is you, then make sure to be aware of your self-talk so that you can encourage it in a healthy direction. Let people see you for who you are, not who you tell them you are, and have peace about the outcome. If your heart is in the right place, it will be obvious.

A smile goes a long way! When you think happy thoughts, that energy becomes apparent in your body language and your facial expressions. Have you ever had a better than average day and found yourself walking through a large group of people, only to receive an unusual amount of smiles greetings and even compliments from total strangers? This happens because people are affected by the energy you give off. When you are happy and friendly, you are radiant, and you attract that energy in return. This type of attractiveness is an excellent area to focus on while you are on your true health journey because it deflects your attention from your superficial traits and causes you to focus on who you really are and how you think.

Buddha Belly doesn't just focus on food and exercise. Gut balancing is just as affected by emotional stresses and negativity. Improving your microbiome will not be achieved if you focus only on what you put in your mouth and ignore what you allow into your head. You must transform from the inside out. Nurturing yourself with love needs to come before the physical changes will take place. Life is really short—too short to self-obsess or focus on things that bring you down. Once you understand this concept, the diet and lifestyle modifications will be easy. Remember to talk yourself up each day. Tell yourself in the mirror that you appreciate your body and what it's done for you, and that from here on out, you will nurture it so that you can enjoy a great quality of life together long into old age.

For information on Gut Health Coaching certification visit hwcacoach.com

CHAPTER 8

Move, Rest, Repeat

A BODY IN motion stays in motion. We are a species that was designed to move. Although the average person knows this, how to go about physical activity can feel daunting. One side of the spectrum touts excessive weight training as the "perfect" mode of health, while the other side pushes you to be the next marathon runner. Physical activity is an enjoyable addition when following *Buddha Belly*'s balancing plan. So, which form of exercise is the way to go?

Honestly, this depends on a few things: where you currently are with fitness, your body type, and, most importantly, what you like! No matter how effective a certain form of exercise may be, if you don't enjoy it, then you won't fully benefit from it. If you are counting down the minutes until it's over, then you won't be truly engaged in your activity causing you not to reap the full rewards. Evaluate where you are at this moment and take into consideration how your body is responding to your new eating habits. Don't be afraid to back off or change direction and follow another mode. Exercise should give you energy, not deplete it. If nothing else, just keep moving. Go for daily walks and stand as much as possible, like when doing computer work. The body is adaptable, and the less time you spend sitting, the more fit you'll be.

How we were designed to move

From the beginning of time, humans were meant to move. With the goal of survival, physical activity usually consisted of a lot of walking, occasional sprinting, climbing, stretching, and lifting. Because so much time was spent out in nature's elements hunting and gathering, this form of cross-training was just a natural part of everyday life. The benefit to this, however, was that it kept the body agile and fit in a way that few gym-goers experience today. The heart and lungs were strong, as was the musculoskeletal frame, and bone density wasn't at all a problem. As with diet, I feel that we perform physical activity too often with the intention of altering our physical body instead of just using it to experience life or increased health. There are those who seek out forms of sports or certain hobbies like rock climbing, strictly for the enjoyment of the activity. These individuals benefit from the lack of stress involved with performing a task out of enjoyment while also experiencing the physical benefits as well.

At one point during my coaching, I did a month of activity that ranged from heavy weights to hill training and basic walking with a stroller. I conducted this experiment over our social media site and titled it "Active April: Throw Away Your Scale." The purpose of this month was to take the focus completely off the dreaded weight tracking and try multiple different forms of activities. I joined a local women's strength training group and practiced high-intensity interval training (HIIT) workouts on the hill by my house, isometric-based DVD's, and even aerial yoga. I liked all of these workouts and was able to note which forms my body responded to best and which ones I enjoyed the most. One of the most enlightening discoveries for me personally was seeing that my body liked many different forms of exercise and possessed almost a need for certain workouts at certain times or on certain days. For instance, at the beginning of the week when I was the most rested, my strength training routine and my HIIT workouts were the most desired and successful. Midweek was an excellent time for yoga and stretching, and daily walking kept me loose. Listening to my body enabled me to give it what it needed and allowed me to appreciate all that it could do.

Although it may be awkward at first, seeing your body move in ways that it hasn't before gives you a new respect for it. Yoga is an excellent example of this. As you improve your practice, your flexibility and form improve. Yoga not only helps you feel peaceful but helps you feel sexy, much like dancing. Yoga is an almost artistic expression and can be done by just about anyone regardless of physical ailments or issues. During the beginning of the Buddha Belly program, you may want to stick to subtle exercises such as yoga, especially if you are new to physical fitness or dealing with adrenal fatigue. This practice is easily tailored to each person no matter where they are while also providing a relaxing experience.

HIIT is a form of burst exercise. Sprinting or heavy lifting (maxing out) for a short hard period of time is an example of HIIT exercise. This type of training is very effective for burning fat and is an efficient way to lean out the body with a short duration of intense activity. Football players practice a lot of HIIT-based workouts. They sprint and tackle full exertion followed by a period of rest before doing this again. Many experts state that this type of fitness is optimal for burning fat and will create the most desirable body.

Strength training is another form of fitness as well as an excellent way to build your musculoskeletal body. As long as proper form is used, isolated movements can be used to build specific muscle groups. This type of exercise is beneficial for the body's metabolic rate (the rate at which it burns energy or calories). The more muscle mass you possess, the more calories you will burn consistently. Strength training can mold the structure of your body and help even extra weight sit more flattering.

Like they say, "Abs are made in the kitchen"

This is true. The majority of physical improvements will become visible with a nurturing form of eating. While fitness has a concrete space in our lives, it is much less effective when the body isn't being fueled and cared for properly. The functions responsible for how your body burns fat and builds muscle vary greatly depending on the level of toxins bogging down your liver. *Buddha Belly* understands the connection between both of these elements, which is why we emphasize the nurturing nutrition portion so strongly.

A great way to look at your body in regard to fitness is like a nice suit or dress. It is something you wear that dresses up what you already have underneath. Despite your body fat percentage, your musculoskeletal frame is your Armani or little black dress. It is a suit designed solely for you and your frame. Performing exercise should firstly be enjoyable, and secondly, it should be a way to tailor that unique outfit to your body. I find that it helps to focus on the body's structure, especially when new to fitness or starting a journey into health. It is far more common to focus on the outer layer of weight or undesirable traits than it is to focus on structure. Again, like with diet, we want to motivate our best self from the inside out, not bully it into existence. Because your body's structure is its support and truest form, focusing on building, stretching, and appreciating it will distract you from negative criticism and allow you to see progress more clearly.

Progress comes in so many forms such as flexibility, speed, heart rate, stamina, strength, agility, and balance. Focus on the positive improvements in these areas while listening to your body's communication. For some people, certain forms of activity such as intense lifting or excessive cardio may not be right for their bodies at a certain point in time. Only perform activities that suit your current state of fitness and progress slowly. Find motivation in everything from improved muscle definition to an increase in stamina. Get creative with your fitness and have solace in the fact that you are already nourishing your body in a new way that is more than half the battle.

You are what you drink

Anyone with a remotely green thumb knows that if you don't water a plant, it will not survive. But before its demise, it will wilt and then slump over before the leaves and petals fall off, and eventually, it will die. Our bodies are approximately sixty percent water. In a day in age where cola and energy drinks are regularly consumed and juice and chocolate milk are considered the "healthy" option, we are very dehydrated. When the body is lacking sufficient H_2O, it can't function as intended. Water is essential for proper digestion, detoxification, and proper vitamin and mineral absorption. When your hydration needs aren't met, symptoms such as fatigue, mood swings, and headache are common, and in severe cases, kidney malfunction and even death can occur. In an already undernourished, overworked population, do we really need to exacerbate our fatigue by ignoring our water needs? It seems ridiculous to me.

In recent studies, it was concluded that approximately seventy-five percent of Americans are chronically dehydrated, and this is largely due to an overconsumption of soda and similar beverages, as well as the lack of whole, fibrous, water-containing foods. Chronic vitamin and mineral deficiencies can come from many things, but chronic dehydration is a significant factor. By staying hydrated, you can eliminate this common cause. It is recommended that the average person consume half of a gallon of water a day. An easy way to achieve this is to limit or omit any non-water-based drinks. Infusing your water with berries and fruit or cucumber is a great way to dress it up. Herbal teas are caffeine-free, and as long as they aren't combined with artificial sweeteners, they are a healthy option as well.

Don't forget your beauty rest

The role that sleep plays in your life cannot be underestimated. Sleep has the ability to make or break you. Believe it or not, the average person needs eight to ten hours of sleep a night to reap the full benefits of bodily rejuvenation. The average adult currently gets around six and a half hours of sleep per night. Children need approximately nine to thirteen hours per night to support healthy growth and brain function. This may sound excessive, but adequate rest is something you need to make time for.

A lot happens during the resting hours. The kidneys and liver work hard to detox that day's exposures, and the digestive system focuses on processing nutrients and repairing its structural integrity and ecosystem. The body works on muscle and tissue repair, memory consolidation, and the functions of hormones that have a multitude of effects on the body. According to the National Sleep Foundation, there are four stages of sleep. Stage one is light sleep or "half-sleep."

Stage two is the onset of sleep where your body temperature drops and your breathing and heart rate become regular. Stages three and four are the stages of deep sleep where the blood pressure drops, breathing slows, muscles relax, hormones are released, and energy is restored. It is during this phase of sleep that your health is most impacted. Interfering with the release of essential hormones has an effect on appetite control, hunger signals, and growth. This can have very negative consequences on a child's development as well as an adult wishing to lose weight and build muscle.

Think of full, complete sleep like a dishwasher or washing machine. If you don't let it finish the cycle, you will likely get dirty dishes or clothes that are too wet to put in the dryer. By repetitively stopping your cycle short, you are inhibiting your body from completing its healthy functions and working against your health goals. Even the important bacteria in your gut rely on your sleep! With gut health being the goal, it is important to prioritize sleep as part of your gut-balancing journey. Scientists are finding that as much as the microbiome affects sleep function, improper sleep also affects the quality and diversity of gut microbes. Gut microbes are like skin cells, constantly dying while the body works to make new ones. Much of this process takes place during sleep, so when adequate sleep is not achieved, it can affect the body's ability to replace the lost microbes.

Sleep is the new Botox!

Just as microbes are replaced during sleep, so are cells. With your skin being the largest organ of the human body, a lot of energy is needed to replace skin cells and repair damage. A lack of rest can age a person very quickly. Studies show accelerated aging of the brain in individuals with poor sleep habits, as well as an increase in Alzheimer's disease. When a person is tired, the body releases more cortisol. The presence of cortisol deteriorates the collagen in the skin, making more lines and wrinkles. We count on the human growth hormones released during rest for strong bones, skin, and muscle mass. Because multiple functions are performed during different stages of sleep, a full cycle of sleep is as crucial to your health as water, diet, and exercise.

REM sleep stands for rapid eye movement. REM sleep should occur for twenty-five of the evening starting about ninety minutes into sleep and occurring every ninety minutes lasting for longer durations as the night goes on. During REM sleep is generally when dreams occur. The brain is active, but the body is limp and possibly "twitchy." Scientists still do not fully understand REM sleep. In one study, when rats were robbed of REM sleep for four weeks, they died. According to an article in *Scientific American*, this could be because REM sleep is needed for regulating body temperature and neurotransmitter levels. They go on to state that "fetuses and babies spend seventy-five percent of their sleeping time in REM." Many psychologists actually have said that they believe that this stage of sleep has a purpose and that it consists of meaningful dreams.

Regardless of the unknown reasons for different stages of sleep, we have enough information to understand the importance of adequate, quality rest. To ignore this area of your health is selling yourself short. As the mother of breastfed babies, I understand that there are forces beyond our control. That is why it is so crucial to make time to rest whenever possible. A midday catnap can do wonders for your energy while helping make up for a night of poor sleep. Setting a "get ready for bed" time is a great way to wind the body down and ensure an earlier shut-eye.

One big disruptor of sleep is technology. Television, computers, phones, and artificial lights keep the body awake. Humans were never designed to live around artificial light. Prehistoric humans would make fire when light was needed and usually slept and woke according to the rise and fall of the sun. Strangely, light from fire does not have the same effect on the brain as artificial illumination. Blue lights and artificial illumination affect our biorhythms, the rhythms that are responsible for our sleep patterns. Too much "light" in the night hours, when the body is trying to wind down, confuses it into thinking that daylight is still present and therefore inhibits the normal rest functions—functions that calm the body and mind, preparing it for restful sleep.

Blue light, or light that is emitted from technological devices, really affects the sleep rhythms and the body's production of melatonin, a hormone responsible for keeping you asleep. In order to set yourself up for sleep success, make it a habit of being in bed by 10 p.m. each night. Most sleep rejuvenation is done between 1 a.m. and 3 a.m. If you are waking during these hours, not only are you not getting restful sleep, but also it is possibly a sign of a bogged-down liver. During these hours is when a large amount of detoxification takes place, and if the liver isn't functioning properly, this could be apparent in the sleep-cycle disruption. Getting to sleep later than 11 p.m. doesn't allow the body to get into the deep sleep necessary for the rejuvenation period by 1 a. m.

Try some of these tips. At least one to two hours before bed, turn off all electronic devices and dim the lights. Try stretching or taking a hot Epsom salt bath to help you relax. Refrain from eating at least three hours before sleep and avoid alcohol. Alcohol is taxing on the liver and actually inhibits restful sleep. Sugar and other stimulants should also be avoided in the evening, and caffeine should be avoided after 10 a.m. For those who suffer from insomnia and chronic fatigue, these avoidances may feel impossible. Relying on a cocktail at night to pass out and stiff coffee throughout the day to keep going is a vicious cycle that only perpetuates a vicious cycle. Sleep issues are a huge sign of a leaky gut. and although these sleep practices may feel difficult at first, they will pay off in the long run. A body and mind that are well rested will reward you with improved mood, hormonal function, and a quality immune system.

Make your bed a spa experience

Instead of looking at sleep as a stressful thing you don't have enough time for or flopping into bed out of exhaustion at the end of the day, make your sleeping environment a peaceful experience. Think of how wonderful it feels to get a good massage. The room is usually dimly lit with low peaceful music or nature sounds and smells of essential oils. Design your bedroom in a way that promotes tranquility. Rub your feet with lavender oil and play some ocean sounds.

Make sure your bed is cozy, and your room is free of clutter. Spend time in your room or bed without technology before actually going to sleep. This is a good place to stretch, meditate, pray, and practice calming your mind. The more you can wind down before actual sleep occurs, the less active your thoughts will become, and the better quality your actual sleep experience will be.

CHAPTER 9

Keeping It Real: Alternative Home and Body Products

HUNDREDS OF THOUSANDS of chemicals have been produced in the last two hundred years, making the full regulation of them almost impossible. The long-term effects of being exposed to all of these toxic substances are still so unknown. Just because the exact effect of any one chemical isn't certain, it is certain that many of these chemicals are responsible for the influx of cancer and other related illness. In one study, scientists found many toxic chemicals present in the DNA of children that were banned decades before the child's conception. This suggests that long after we "clean up the problem," these toxic substances are still saturated in our environment, only left to harm future generations.

Nonorganic methods of growing food have also poisoned our food and our environment. If you have ever watched a small prop plane spray pesticides over a field of corn, you can imagine the quantity of toxic chemicals present in our air, doused on our food, and left to seep into our groundwater. Buying organic whenever possible, especially when purchasing fruits and veggies, will help lessen your exposure. Buying directly from a local organic farmer is even better. Local organic produce is the next best thing to growing your own food. It allows you to consume food shortly after it is harvested, and most operations will be happy to give you a tour of their farm and let you see for yourself how the food is grown and treated.

What good is a clean toilet if it gives you a weak gut?

Household cleaners, chemicals, and beauty products are crammed into most cupboards. There are specific products for everything. One product is for the toilet, the other is for the sink, and then there is the floor cleaner that might be next to the glass spray—each individual concoction promising to help make your life easier and your home spotless. What these products fail to mention is that along with a squeaky-clean countertop, you will also be exposed to a long list of chemicals and their side effects.

The most toxic chemicals found in the average home consist of anticorrosive products: oven cleaners and toilet cleaners. Although these are the highest toxicity, it's the everyday "low toxicity" products that add up over time. Because these low-toxicity products are used so frequently, the low levels of chemicals build up in the body. Then there's the fact that multiple different products contain the same chemicals, so in one day, you are easily exposed to these toxic substances again and again.

Some concerning ingredients found in everyday products (mainly body products) are parabens, which are a form of preservative used to prevent bacterial growth. Parabens mimic estrogen and have been found in breast cancer tumors. They are currently used in many different products but are very common in beauty products and shampoos. Phytates are used to create flexibility in plastic substances and are linked to endocrine disruption and cancer. Triclosan is another ingredient used as an antimicrobial in soap products that is another endocrine disruptor, especially affecting the thyroid and reproductive organs.

Sodium lauryl sulfate (SLS) is the ingredient that causes foaming in soaps. The scary truth behind SLS is that it can mix with other chemicals causing severe kidney and respiratory issues, as well as hormone disruptions. Hormone disruptors interfere with the body's chemical messaging by blocking or mimicking natural hormonal actions. The more you dig into ingredient labels of common household cleaning and personal care products, the longer the toxic

BUDDHA BELLY

list will be. Ironically, basic soap and water clean just as effectively as their health-damaging counterparts.

Antiperspirants in deodorants contain aluminum. Antiperspirant means "no sweat," and blocking your sweat glands with aluminum is how this is achieved. Keep in mind that your sweat glands are meant as an exit for waste. The usage of antiperspirants is strongly linked to breast cancer. The correlation between antiperspirants and breast cancer is higher among women because women generally shave their armpits, thus opening the pores to absorbing more of these chemicals than a man's hairy armpit would. Add to that the fact that the detoxification outlet is being blocked by the aluminum, keeping the waste stagnant within the body, and it becomes apparent as to why we need to change our ways with deodorizing.

Much like foods, our environment has become so tainted with chemicals that it can seem impossible to avoid them. It is impossible to completely avoid all these substances because they are present in the air and water, as well as in building materials and fabrics. The good news is that we can make a significant impact on our health and our levels of exposure by making clean pure choices wherever possible. *Buddha Belly* has included some of our favorite DIY recipes for some common body and cleaning products. There are many more natural options than what is in this chapter, but we have shared some of the most important substitutions that happen to be very effective and easy to make.

Pure body products

> *Deodorant*
> ¼ c. coconut oil melted
> ¼ c. cornstarch
> ¼ c. baking soda
> 10 drops desired essential oil
>
> Mix all ingredients until it forms a paste. Pour the paste into the desired jar or tin and refrigerate for an hour to solidify. The mixture will vary

73

inconsistently depending on temperature, so we recommend keeping in a sealed container for warm climates and situations.

Face wash
3 tbs. coconut oil, melted
3 tbs. baking soda
5 drops of desired essential oil

Combine all ingredients and keep in a small container. If the mixture gets too solid, just rub between palms until it forms a cream consistently, and rinse after use. Larger batches can be made after you gauge how much will be used before ingredients will expire.

Sweet body scrub
1 c. coconut oil
½ c. brown sugar
3 tbs. ground cinnamon

Melt coconut oil, but do not heat it up. Next, add the other two ingredients and mix to form a sandy consistency. Store in a jar and use it as an exfoliant. Rinse when done.

Body whipped cream
1 c. solid coconut oil
20 drops chosen essential oil

Add solid coconut oil and essential oil to a bowl and mix on medium-high for 6–7 minutes until it forms a thick whip. Store in a closed container and use it in place of body lotions.

Mineralizing toothpaste
3 tbs. coconut oil
3 tbs. pink Himalayan sea salt
3 tbs. baking soda
10 drops peppermint essential oil

Melt coconut oil and mix in other ingredients. Keep the mixture in a jar and spoon out for each use.

Bug repellent
4 oz. witch hazel
4 oz. distilled water
25 drops tea tree oil
25 drops eucalyptus oil

Mix all ingredients and put in a glass spray bottle, or divide between multiple small bottles.

Home products

Glass cleaner
¼ c. distilled water
¼ c. vinegar
5 drops chosen essential oil

Mix all ingredients together and keep in a glass jar or glass spray bottle. Avoid plastic containers and store labeled in the fridge.

Surface grime cleaner
½ c. vegetable oil
1 c. baking soda

Mix the two ingredients together to form a paste and scrub into grimy areas with a sponge. Rinse when finished.

Laundry detergent
2 lb. baking soda
12 oz. Epsom salts
2 lb. washing soda
1 (4 oz.) bar castle soap
1.5 containers of OxiClean Baby

Mix all ingredients and store in a glass container. Use about 2 tablespoons per large load. Adjust if necessary.

Toilet bowl discs
1.5 c. baking soda
½ c. lemon juice
25 drops lemon essential oil

Mix all ingredients together and divide into cupcake tins. Let sit until dry. Once dry, store in bags and use one in the back of the toilet (in the tank) when needed.

Floor cleaner
1 c. white vinegar
1 tbs. liquid castle soap
1 c. baking soda
10 drops essential oil
2 gal. tap water

Mix all ingredients into a mop bucket; stir until baking soda dissolve. Warm water will help this process. Use on floors and discard when finished.

CHAPTER 10

Probiotics and Super Healing Foods

THINK OF THE little microorganisms in your body like little fish in a fish tank. I am not an expert on fish or fish tanks, but I feel confident enough to use this analogy. A fish tank is its own little ecosystem. If you fill it with the right variety of fish, clean it regularly, and plant the right plants, the water should stay clean enough to provide the oxygen necessary for the fish's survival. With that said, the fish still need to eat, so you must feed them accordingly. Failing to do this will starve the fish to death and throw off the balance of the tank. Assuming the tank has a variety of fish, such as bottom feeders who clean the muck off the bottom of the tank, you can see why the loss of this life would interfere with the function of the tank. On top of this, you lose fish every day to old age.

Your body is like the fish tank with the bacteria in your gut and throughout your body being the fish. Like the fish, the bacteria need to eat to be strong. If they are not fed, then they become weak and will not optimally contribute to the ecosystem of the tank. When fish are lost, new ones also need to be added to the tank in order to maintain balance. So, if your body is like the tank and your microbiome is the fish, then what is the fish food?

Prebiotics (not to be confused with probiotics) are what feed the microbiome. They are your fish food. Prebiotics are plant fibers that the body can't digest. It instead saves these nutrients for the gut bacteria to feed on. Prebiotics are found in whole foods such as fruits, vegetables, garlic, onions, and other plant-based foods. Consuming an adequate amount of healthy plant foods is very essential to maintaining the health of your gut bacteria. This is easily done following the Buddha Belly eating plan.

Now! Let's go back to probiotics, or your "fish." Probiotics need to be replenished frequently. How we can go about doing that is by taking an oral supplement and consuming probiotic fermented foods. While supplemental probiotics are part of the Buddha Belly protocol, relying on supplement form alone isn't necessarily enough. Probiotics are very sensitive and often can be killed off in the stomach acid or by heat, before ever reaching their destination in the gut. Another challenge to probiotics in supplemental form is that scientists still don't know exactly which bacteria benefit which people. Because there are so many strains and the need for different strains differ from person to person, it is currently impossible to make a supplement that will benefit all persons. This is why *Buddha Belly* recommends a multistrain that contains *Lactobacillus bifidus* and *L. acidophilus* since these are the strains known to support digestive health in general. Also, look for enteric-coated capsules that have a strong coating to withstand stomach acid, as well as a supplement that is non-GMO and preferably raw. Avoid the brands that contain sugar in their probiotics. This should be listed in the ingredients list.

Aside from using supplemental forms of probiotics, we can benefit from consuming probiotics in the form of natural foods. Foods that have been fermented to some degree will contain natural probiotics. *Buddha Belly* advocates natural sources whenever possible. Nature knows more about what our bodies need than science ever will, and focusing on natural sources of probiotics in foods is an efficient way to let nature suggest the adequate combination of bacteria. Raw versions of kefir, kombucha, yogurt, sauerkraut, aged cheeses, sourdough, beer, wine, and vinegar are all-natural sources of probiotics. Since *Buddha Belly* excludes dairy, alcohol, and wheat during the first phase, we have emphasized alternative food sources of probiotics and have included recipes for these. This will allow you to incorporate them into your health regimen and maximize the opportunity to strengthen your microbiome.

Kefir

Kefir is a yogurt-like drink, originally made by adding cultured "grains" to milk. These cultures are made of yeast and lactic acid. The cultures feed on the milk sugars causing them to ferment. The process takes about 24 hours. When making dairy kefir, raw organic milk should be used. Even those with lactose intolerance may be able to tolerate milk in raw form, especially once fermented. If you really don't do well with cow's milk, raw goat's milk has smaller lactose molecules and is even easier on digestion. Although milk kefir is superior to any other form of kefir, during the first phase of Buddha Belly, we recommend coconut milk kefir. Although it doesn't possess the strength of milk kefir, it will provide many of the same benefits while you are healing your gut enough to reintroduce raw dairy products.

Recipe (coconut milk):

2 tbs. kefir grains
2 c. canned organic coconut milk
2 c. regular unsweetened organic coconut milk
Glass jar
Mesh cloth

Combine coconut milk in the glass jar and add the kefir grains. Cover with mesh using a rubber band and set in a warm place for 24 hours. After 12 hours, stir the mixture well. After the 24-hour fermentation period, strain the kefir through a fine strainer and keep in the fridge for up to a week. Save the grains in a glass jar in the fridge for later use. The mixture will smell like yeast. You can add vanilla for flavor or a small amount of maple syrup, but we recommend adding this individually before consumption since sugar can negatively impact the grains.

Kombucha

Kombucha is a drink made from tea and using a yeast-bacteria SCOBY, or starter. The starter feeds off the sugar in the sweet tea causing fermentation. Kombucha isn't as potent in beneficial bacteria as kefir, but still provides health benefits. The yeast causes an almost carbonated effect. Kefir can be made from any kind of tea, but we recommend an organic tea, free of chemicals. Black varieties are commonly used to make kombucha. Small amounts of kombucha are allowed in all phases of the Buddha Belly protocol.

Recipe:

15 c. filtered water
1 c. sugar
10 teaspoons loose leaf tea or 10 tea bags
2 tbs. apple cider vinegar with the mother
½ gal. Mason jar
Coffee filter

Start by bringing the water to a boil in a pot. Add in the tea and let steep for 10 minutes. Stir in sugar until it dissolves; then filter the tea and pour it into the Mason jar. Add the vinegar and the SCOBY to the jar and cover the top using the coffee filter and securing it with a rubber band. Let sit in a warm dark place for 5–30 days. Once you smell a sour odor, you know the process is working, and you can taste test it to reach your desired level of fermentation. Once the kombucha is where you would like it, transfer it to separate bottles and leave bottles at room temperature for a few days to add extra carbonation. The remaining SCOBY should be divided into two parts: the main mother SCOBY (your starter) and the "baby" that grew off of it. Keep these in glass jars submerged in a little kombucha liquid, in your fridge, covered for later use.

Buddha Belly puts a strong emphasis on the consumption of fermented foods. Kifer is a powerhouse of probiotics, and kombucha is an enjoyable alternative to sodas and juices while adding healthy bacteria. Aside from these two drinks, you can get probiotics from fermented foods like sauerkraut, kimchi, and pickles. We recommend making your own or purchasing organic varieties that don't use artificial chemicals, sugar, and dyes. An easy way to add more good bacteria to your gut is by consuming organic apple cider vinegar with the mother. The "mother" is the active culture present in vinegar that is responsible for its probiotic content. Apple cider vinegar can be used for everything from stomach aches to cleaning. I even used it to remove a wart my son had! If it is too strong for you to shoot straight, you can dilute it with some water. I recommend two tablespoons first thing in the morning.

Homemade sauerkraut

Raw sauerkraut purchased in the store is rather costly, and it's honestly such an easy thing to make at home! You will need the following:

½ gal. Mason jar
1 medium head of cabbage
1 tbs. sea salt
Canning weight

Start by washing the mason jar very well to avoid bacteria and let dry completely. Next chop up a medium head of cabbage into small strands, usually larger than typical commercial sauerkraut. In a large glass or stainless bowl, add the sea salt to the cabbage. Toss it around a bit and then massage it in with your clean hands. You will feel the cabbage wilt a bit as it breaks down, which you want it to do. You can also add peppers to spice it up or spices like coriander if you choose. Next, pack the half-gallon jar with the cabbage until it is about two inches from the top of the jar. Fill the jar with purified water just until the cabbage is covered. You will want to be able to fit the canning weight on top to hold the cabbage below the water. Failure to do so can cause your cabbage to float above the water line and collect mold. Mold will contaminate the entire batch so a canning weight is an essential tool. You will want to keep the mixture away from the lid also. Let the sauerkraut sit at room temperature for 10–20 days. You will want to burp it every day or two. To burp the sauerkraut, just unscrew the lid a bit to release the pressure, or else, too much pressure will build up and can explode your glass jar. Taste it after about 10 days and determine if you'd like it to ferment longer. Once it is where you want it, you can store it in the fridge. Research the shelf life in your area.

What's all the hype about bone broth?

Bone broth is a substance resulting from cooking the marrow and cartilage out of meat, bones, and ligaments. At a cool temperature, it is like a jelly and when heated turns to liquid. Bone broth was originally the way people made soups and stews and maximized all of the animals that they killed for nutrition purposes. Nowadays, you can buy different stock from chicken to beef, but it is mainly flavored with MSG (a very unhealthy salt additive), other fillers, and artificial flavors.

Real wholesome bone broth can easily be made at home and is an excellent complement to the Buddha Belly regimen. Bone broth is high in collagen, which helps the elasticity of the skin. The lack of elasticity in our skin is what contributes to sag, wrinkles, and cellulite. Bone broth is also high in glucosamine, which not only helps joint pain and function but also can help restore a leaky gut. As stated before, leaky gut is a condition where there are large openings present in the lining of the intestines, and in order to help these junctions tighten, we need to cultivate a healthy bacterial presence and feed the body nutrients for proper tissue repair—hence, glucosamine, which can also be taken in the form of a supplement—but like all things, the natural form is recommended as an easier and gentler way to get this hearty nutrient.

Bone broth is rich in many vitamins and minerals, phosphorus, calcium, and magnesium, which are present in the bones and marrow and are cooked out into a liquid form that surpasses any supplement. They contribute to joint and bone health, as well as an increased immune system. These are just some of the reasons why bone broth is being hailed as a "superfood." The benefits of it are pretty super, and unlike supplemental L-glutamine, anyone can consume it—pregnant or nursing women, and anyone can use it, such as pregnant or nursing women. It is very important to remember to acquire the bones through a healthy source. Organic grass-fed or wild animal bones are best. Anything the animal comes in contact with through diet and environment will be found inside their tissues, so unless you want to drink concentrated amounts of chemicals, antibiotics, and junk with your broth, then make sure the source is clean. Although bone broth can be made in different ways, we have included a tried and true version that we have found to have the best results.

Bone broth in the slow cooker

Bones from grass-finished chicken or beef (enough to fit in your slow cooker)
2 tbs. organic apple cider vinegar
½ c. onion
2 cloves organic garlic
1 tbs. pink Himalayan sea salt (optional)

Roast bones in the oven at 400 degrees for 30 minutes if raw (optional). Place bones in a Crock-Pot and add enough water just to cover. Cook on low for twelve hours. Add remaining ingredients and cook for another twelve hours. Strain and place in the fridge. When the mixture cools, remove fat off the top and use or freeze within three days.

Instant Pot (updated)

When I originally wrote this recipe section in 2015, I had not yet been introduced to the magnificence of the Instant Pot, a tool capable of cutting my cooking time down to a fraction. Using the Instant Pot to make bone broth is initially just like the crock. You will add all the ingredients, cover just over the bones with water, and instead of cooking for 24 hours, 2 hours on high will do the trick! Release manually and voilà! Bone broth should be a staple of your gut health lifestyle.

CHAPTER 11

Eating and Healing in Three Phases

BY THIS POINT in your Buddha Belly journey, I hope you feel enlightened about new information and motivated to do things differently than you have before. This is the exciting part of the process! Making strict dietary changes can be very overwhelming, so during this time, there are a few things to keep in mind.

Once the sugar is out, your ability to adhere to a new way of eating will become so much easier. Sugar is said to be four times as addictive as cocaine, and anyone with a sweet tooth can see why. It is in the majority of processed foods keeping your body suffering and addicted. By following the elimination portion, you will rid your body of the intense cravings through stabilizing blood sugars and removing chemicalized forms of sugar from your body.

When all else fails, meditate. If stress is getting the better part of you, stop what you're doing and practice breathing and calming your mind. Schedule this time every day, more than once if necessary.

Just keep moving. Walk. Dance. Do yoga. Whatever you do, just don't stop moving within a healthy degree. This will keep your mood strong and distract you from your thoughts about food while detoxing.

You are not dieting! Nurturing your body into a state of health and well-being is like chicken soup when you are sick. It is a way to nourish yourself so that you get back to great.

Enjoy your accomplishments. Don't stress the distance in front of you. Enjoy the present moment. You own *this* moment, and that's all you need to focus on.

Pretty soon, you'll wake up and wonder why you ever thought you couldn't do this. That day is just around the corner.

Rather than focus on what not to eat, let's start with what foods to eat!

Foods to focus on

Vegetables. The presence of veggies is the one commonality in the majority of "diets," and so it should be. Vegetables, especially raw greens, will provide you immense fiber and nutrition, as well as bulk to fill up your belly, leaving you satisfied and full of energy after meals.

Wild, grass-fed animal products. Organic animals that have lived on their natural diet are the best form of nutrition for healing your gut. A majority of the meat, eggs, and dairy in the United States are factory farmed. These animals are inoculated with numerous antibiotics and hormones. They are also kept in confined spaces and fed GMO corn and soy-based foods that their bodies were never intended to consume. Because of this, their meat and by-products are chemically tainted, are high in omega-6 fats, and carry a much greater risk of salmonella. *Buddha Belly* does not advocate basing your meals around animal products; however, we have found a moderate amount to be highly valuable in the process of gut healing because of the need for collagen in tissue repair. Look for grass-finished organic meats and eggs. Wild game is even better.

Organic fruits. Eating organic fruits in moderation will help fuel your carbohydrate intake as well as provide vitamins and minerals. Do not consume fruits in the form of juice as this is lacking fiber and will raise blood sugars too fast. Organic berries are a perfect low-glycemic option and are high in antioxidants.

Healthy fats. Balanced amounts of healthy fats such as olive oil, coconut oil, and avocado and avocado oil are a welcomed addition to Buddha Belly's focus plan. These fats will provide you with energy as well as nutrition while soothing your gut.

Nuts and seeds. With the exception of peanuts, which are actually a legume, nuts and seeds consumed in moderate amounts are allowed during this process and will benefit you much like healthy oils, by providing fats and essential nutrients. Quinoa, although similar to a grain, is actually a seed and in small amounts is fine. Those with certain conditions such as diverticulitis should avoid nuts and seeds, but most others will be fine with small amounts intermixed throughout their diet.

Organic potatoes. Small amounts of potatoes will provide a nutritious source of carbohydrates and fiber. We advocate sweet potatoes over white varieties due to their low glycemic index. For those with insulin sensitivity, be mindful not to overconsume potatoes. Instead, rely more on vegetables and quinoa for your carbohydrates.

Recommended supplements for the first thirty days: A multistrain quality probiotic, vitamin D, magnesium, and digestive enzymes for main meals to aid in digestion, quality grass-fed collagen protein to assist in intestinal tissue repair, smoothie in breakfast, and bone broth (consumed at least three times a week and up to seven times weekly).

See buddhabellycoach.com for available supplements or ask your local provider.

As with everything Buddha Belly preaches, listen to your body. If you have consistent adverse reactions to any of these suggested foods, avoid them for the first thirty days and then try them again during the reintroduction phase.

Phase 1: The first thirty days

The purpose of the first thirty days is to remove foods from the diet that are common allergens and gut irritants, as well as processed nonfoods. One reason for this is to allow the gut to begin to heal while focusing on recolonizing the probiotic bacteria. The other purpose of the first thirty days is to detox the body from addictive substances such as refined sugars, processed foods, and alcohol so that a nurturing diet becomes easier.

Depending on where your current dietary habits are and what level of toxin buildup exists in your body, you may experience a variety of symptoms. It is common when detoxing to experience cold-like symptoms as well as intestinal changes. If you experience intestinal changes that remain after a couple of days or are associated with specific foods, consider that it could be that food triggering an unpleasant response and remove it for the time being. Headaches are also common, as are mood swings. These are especially present in those coming off of refined sugars and caffeine. Herbal teas and the use of essential oils can help lessen the discomfort of these withdrawal symptoms. While these are common detox symptoms, remember to always consult your physician before beginning any dietary regimen.

During this period, physical activity is important and can alleviate discomfort and redirect energy. It is important to remember to listen to your body and not overdo it. Even basic walking is a practice that can be incorporated into your daily schedule and extended as your body becomes more capable. Adequate rest will allow your body to rejuvenate and rebuild, which is the point of this month. There will be no cookie-cutter experience for everyone as everybody is different. It is your job to listen to yours and nurture it accordingly. We will go into more on how to listen to your body in the next chapter.

Habits for the first thirty days

Include the following:

Probiotic. Take quality probiotic daily.

Breakfast. Drink your breakfast (healthy smoothy recipe including grass-fed collagen protein) or chia pudding.

Snacks. Eat superfood snacks (two to three a day, recipes in back).

Vegetables. Fill half your plate with veggies for both lunch and dinner (focus on mostly raw greens).

Rest. Let your digestion rest for twelve to sixteen hours each night (e.g., 7 p.m.–7 a.m.)

Fermentation. Eat fermented food or beverage daily

Eliminate the following:

Processed foods and beverages. Almost anything that requires an ingredient label is a processed food. Processed foods have a high concentration of chemicals, preservatives, refined sugars, and unhealthy fats. Eliminating these foods is crucial to healing your gut.

Dairy products. Most dairy comes from cows that are fed growth hormones and excessive antibiotics. On top of this, the pasteurization process renders the lactose hard to digest and lacking nutrients. Avoid all dairy for the first thirty days. After this point, you can experiment with raw organic and fermented dairy.

Wheat, flours, and gluten. Gluten is very hard on digestion. Many of the varieties of wheat are genetically modified or have come in contact with GMOs. You will likely see substantial improvement in your symptoms by eliminating gluten.

Refined sugars. Cane sugars, sugar syrups, and flavorings are all forms of refined sugars. Eliminating processed foods and avoiding adding table sugar to foods will help eliminate their consumption. If you desire some sugar (provided you don't have insulin issues), use a small amount of real maple syrup or raw honey. *Buddha Belly* has provided some yummy sweet options in the back—the recipe portion of this book.

Grains. With the exception of small amounts of quinoa, which is actually a seed, we have eliminated grains during the first phase because whole healthy grains also come with the downside of being high in antinutrients or phytates. The phytate in grains is reduced when soaked, sprouted, or cooked, but the high carbohydrate content that does feed good bacteria also feeds the bad. Until your gut microbes are balanced, it is best to keep grains out. After the first phase, occasional small amounts of whole grains may be consumed if soaked and prepared properly.

Peanuts, beans, and legumes. A lot of people have a hard time tolerating the gastrointestinal effects of beans and legumes. Along with their susceptibility to carry molds, beans are high in antinutrients and can be very hard on the digestive system. During the healing process, it is important to keep these out of your diet until the gut feels healed enough to experiment with them in small amounts.

Corn. Corn and the products made from it should be strictly avoided during the initial phase. Corn can be just as hard if not harder on the gut than gluten, and much of it is genetically modified. After the first phase, you can experiment with small amounts of organic, non-GMO varieties. Avoid all products made from corn such as cornmeal, corn syrup, cornstarch, and corn oil.

Soy. Most soy in the United States is also genetically modified. On top of that, soy can disrupt healthy hormonal function. It is especially detrimental to those with a thyroid disorder. Soy should be avoided in all forms: edamame, soy sauce, soy lecithin, and soy milk. Soy can come in a multitude of forms and names, so eliminating processed foods will make it easier to avoid. For those who do not suffer from an adrenal or thyroid disorder, small occasional amounts of organic fermented soy may be experimented with after the first sixty days but shouldn't be used as a main source of protein.

Caffeine. Caffeine is very hard on adrenal function and sometimes on blood sugars. We recommend eliminating caffeine in general. Small amounts of organic green tea can provide a nutritious, less acidic alternative while detoxing. If you absolutely can't go without coffee, try one c. of organic half-decaf coffee in the morning.

Alcohol. Alcohol suppresses the immune system and slows the body's metabolic rate (fat burning). Many forms of beers and beverages are also made with high-fructose corn syrups and chemicals, as well as being high in gluten. Alcohol also disrupts quality, healing sleep. In moderation, healthy alcohol options can have a place in your life after the first thirty days. During the reintroduction phase, we will discuss how to choose clean drink options without backpedaling on your gut's progress.

Phase 2: Reintroduction (thirty days)

After the first thirty days, you can start reintroducing small amounts of certain whole foods to your gut. If you have a severe case of leaky gut and autoimmune issues, you may want to extend the first phase longer than thirty days. The foods to experiment with during this phase are raw organic dairy, organic non-GMO corn, whole gluten-free grains, and clean alcoholic beverages. Due to their negative effects on gut healing, addiction level, and/or the lack of nutrients, we recommend leaving refined sugars, processed foods, gluten, excessive caffeine, and soy out of your diet still at this point.

Wait at least seventy-two hours between food introductions and only add one at a time. Intolerant reactions can wait a day or two before showing up, so in order to eliminate confusion, focus on one at a time.

When experimenting with the reintroduction of foods during this phase, it is important to journal when you add something back. This will allow you to be aware of which foods your body doesn't respond well to. If you have a negative reaction to a particular food or substance, that is a good indication that that food or substance has damaged and possibly still will damage your gut. You will be able to use this information to make choices in the future regarding what you consume and how often.

Alcohol should be reintroduced in the same way as foods, not within a seventy-two-hour period of any other reintroduced food. You should also choose varieties that are clean such as organic red wine and clean (unsweetened) clear liquor, such as vodka. Organic craft beers may be tried after this month if your body responds well to wheat.

Phase 3: Developing a Buddha Belly way of life

After putting in a strict and progressive sixty days, you will have likely noticed some amazing things about your body, as well as your thoughts and feelings. Depending on how severe your issues were when starting this, your body may continue to improve. For others, you will want to maintain the YOU that you have nurtured into being. Here are a few tips:

Continue to build your meals around vegetables, making this the center stage.

Choose organic, properly sourced and fed animal products, fruits, and veggies.

Keep GMOs and processed foods out of your diet as much as possible, along with unhealthy fats. Refined sugar is especially addictive and can be easily substituted with natural sweeteners like raw honey and real maple syrup.

Make probiotic-rich, fermented foods a consistent part of your diet.

Limit your intake of whole grains, corn, and beans, and when consuming them, prepare them properly by soaking and sprouting prior to cooking.

Choose raw, unpasteurized, organic dairy products.

Remember what foods interfere with your body and your gut's homeostasis, and if you must consume these foods, save them for a rare occasion.

Never quit moving, meditating, and loving yourself!

A "baby step" approach

Buddha Belly was written to share the culmination of information that has come to be at this place in time, along with over a decade of my personal education and experiences. Combining holistic health along with the experiences of many contributing individuals, it was my intention to write a book that consisted of all this information in hopes that it would touch a lot of people. With that said, there are people, including those I have worked with, who may feel overwhelmed to tackle *Buddha Belly's* full sixty-day process at once. Because of this, *Buddha Belly* has included a "baby step" approach so that everyone can use this information to start progressing their health and defying the current rate of disease. In the long run, you will all reach the finish line.

You can still follow the focus portion of the main protocol. Drinking your breakfast in the form of a healthy smoothie, consuming large amounts of mainly raw veggies with your large meals, and adding the listed supplements will naturally add nutrition as well as gut-healing benefits.

First thirty days

For the initial phase of the baby-step process, we have chosen to eliminate the substances that are consistently hard on the body:

Gluten

Corn

Artificial sweeteners

For this period, you will want to avoid anything with wheat or any form of gluten present in it, all corn products, and any artificial sugars.

Practice the mind-body-soul suggestions listed in the book. Relax, get adequate sleep, and focus on positive thoughts and affirmations.

Days 31–60

At this time, you should have already noticed improvements by removing gluten, corn, and artificial sweeteners. The next step is assuring that your diet consists of only whole foods. Pulling the foods listed below out of your diet will help achieve this:

Soy

Refined sugars

Unhealthy fats

Processed foods

Alcohol

By the end of this phase, you should see substantial improvements in your body and your health. Your cravings should start to become mild and easily satisfied in healthier ways.

Days 61–90

At this point in the baby-step approach, your body is ready to pull some commonly irritating and allergenic foods. Below we have given you a list of the recommended foods to remove for the next thirty days, in order to allow more intense healing of the gut:

Grains (except quinoa)

Dairy

Beans, legumes, and peanuts

Caffeine

By the end of this phase, your gut should be significantly improved, and you will be ready to experiment with reintroduction.

Reintroduction: Days 91–120

Follow the reintroduction and maintenance approach on previous pages.

CHAPTER 12

Hacking Your Own Gut Journal

Loving your body with food

BUDDHA BELLY WAS written for the purpose of facilitating health through mind, body, and soul. The main component of physical health is the health of your microbiome or "gut." Through *Buddha Belly*'s elimination phase, focusing on life-giving foods is essential. A diet high in fresh organic vegetables and some fruits will keep the PH of the body in a more alkaline state, making it an undesirable environment for disease. Complementing fresh produce with clean morally and healthily raised protein will nourish your body in a new way. Eating in a nurturing way not only is healing for the body and the gut but also with the right recipes can be a beautiful and satisfying experience. In the last chapter, we have included some of our favorite Buddha Belly-approved recipes that are excellent for all phases of your health journey. For more fun demos, blog content, supplements, and recipes, check out buddhabellycoach.com.

Throughout this chapter, you will be able to use these pages as a done-for-you journal and a quick-reference shopping list. We have broken down the step-by-step process of journaling through the elimination phase and the reintroduction phase, using the body's signals to guide the way. Below we have listed some of the common signs and symptoms that the body is signaling an issue with a specific food. Read through these signals and start your own process utilizing the journaling pages in this chapter and the recipes in Chapter 13.

Listening to your body's cues

Common signals that the body is having an intolerant response include the following:

Digestive issues. Gas, bloating, irregular elimination patterns, heartburn, and stomach upset are some examples. After feeling "clean and lean" during the elimination portion, it will become much more obvious to you when your digestive system is acting out like a toddler throwing a temper tantrum, ranging from mild bloating to full-blown intestinal anarchy!

Skin changes. Acne, dryness, rashes, and eczema are common to see. The skin is the body's largest organ, and all organs are affected by a leaky gut. You just so happen to wear this particular organ across your face, so read it like a book! Often psoriasis and eczema are directly related to gluten intolerance. I have known a few parents who have removed this one substance from their children's foods and watched their skin abrasions disappear.

Mood changes. This one is huge for me. Years ago, after a month without any alcohol whatsoever, I chose to drink one beer—just one. That was a bad choice not only due to the sugar and chemical content but also due to the high concentration of wheat. For two solid days, I felt incredibly agitated and restless and couldn't figure out why. That's where journaling comes in handy because that one beer was the only thing I had done differently in a month.

Energy. Feeling lethargic, exhausted, or even manic are notable bodily communication. If you throw the wrong oil in your car, you can expect it not to run right and probably sound kind of funny too. You are your best machine. If you aren't running right, then you possibly filled your tank with the wrong fuel.

Headaches and pains. We get too used to popping a pill at the first sign of a pounding head without considering the cause. My husband's headaches usually mean one of four things: He hasn't drunk enough water, his spine is out, he's lacking sleep, or he ate something he shouldn't have. Achy and stiff joints can signal intolerance as well, so if you go from feeling pretty agile to creeping out of bed like you need a walker, food could be the cause.

Allergy-like/cold symptoms. Watery eyes, stuffy nose, and a dry irritated throat are things to be aware of. Environmental toxins can produce reactivity like this too, so do note if you have come into contact with any harsh cleaning agents, fertilizers, or body products.

Water retention, swelling, and puffiness. Different things may cause you to retain water. If you notice a difference in the fit of your clothing overnight or a noticeable puffiness under your eyes or in your face, hands, or legs, consider what you have consumed. Fluctuations can occur due to things such as hormones and salt intake as well, but after a while, you will know your body enough to decipher the reason for these symptoms.

Focus Food List

INCLUDING BUT NOT limited to

Greens

Alfalfa sprouts, arugula, asparagus, basil, bean sprouts, bok choy, broccoli, butter lettuce, cabbage, celery, cucumber, collard greens, dandelion greens, fennel, green beans, kale, kelp, leafy greens, leeks, lemon grass, lettuce, mustard greens, parsley, spinach, watercress, and Zucchini

Colored veggies

Bell pepper, cauliflower, cherry tomatoes, chili peppers, eggplant, garlic, ginger, green peppers, jalapeno, mushrooms, okra, onions, red bell pepper, tomatillo, tomatoes, and water chestnuts

Starches and gluten-free grains

Banana squash, beets, butternut squash, carrots, potatoes, pumpkins, squash, sweet potatoes, and quinoa

Healthy fats

Avocado, avocado oil, coconut oil, ghee, grass-fed butter, olives, olive oil, and sesame oil

Nuts and seeds

Almonds, brazil nuts, chia seeds, hazelnuts, macadamia nuts, pecans, pistachio, sesame, sunflower seeds, and walnuts

Animal proteins

Eggs, meats, and seafood, preferably organic, grass-finished, wild-caught, and wild-game ones

Fermented foods

Kefir, kimchi, kombucha, miso, pickles, sauerkraut, vinegar

Journaling
The Elimination Phase

THE CURRENT STATE of my wellness rated 1–10 (10 being great and 1 being terrible)

Weight:
Mood:
Skin:
Digestion:
Sleep:
Energy:
Focus:
Joint health:
Muscle strength:
Headaches:
Cycle regularity:
PMS:
Libido:
Food cravings:
Elimination regularity:

Food Eliminated:
Date:

Food Eliminated:
Date:

Food eliminated:
Date:

Food eliminated:
Date:

Food Eliminated:
Date:

Food Eliminated:
Date:

Thirty-Day Elimination Journal

Week 1

How I feel

_____
_____
_____
_____

Thoughts

_____
_____
_____
_____

My body

_____
_____
_____
_____

I AM focus

_____
_____
_____
_____

My stress strategy

_____
_____
_____
_____

My fitness

_____
_____
_____
_____

Journaling notes

_____
_____
_____
_____
_____
_____
_____
_____
_____
_____
_____

Thirty-Day Elimination Journal

Week 2

How I feel

_____
_____
_____
_____

Thoughts

_____
_____
_____
_____

My body

_____
_____
_____
_____

I AM focus

_____
_____
_____
_____

My stress strategy

_____
_____
_____
_____

My fitness

_____
_____
_____
_____

Journaling notes

_____
_____
_____
_____
_____
_____
_____
_____
_____
_____
_____

Thirty-Day Elimination Journal

Week 3

How I feel

_____
_____
_____
_____

Thoughts

_____
_____
_____
_____

My body

_____
_____
_____
_____

I AM focus

_____
_____
_____
_____

My stress strategy

_____
_____
_____
_____

My fitness

_____
_____
_____
_____

Journaling notes

_____
_____
_____
_____
_____
_____
_____
_____
_____
_____
_____

Thirty-Day Elimination Journal

Week 4

How I feel

_____
_____
_____
_____

Thoughts

_____
_____
_____
_____

My body

_____
_____
_____
_____

I AM focus

_____
_____
_____
_____

My stress strategy

_____
_____
_____
_____

My fitness

_____

_____

_____

_____

Journaling notes

_____

_____

_____

_____

_____

_____

_____

_____

_____

_____

Journaling
The Reintroduction Phase

THE CURRENT STATE of my wellness rated 1–10 (10 being great and 1 being terrible)

Weight:
Mood:
Skin:
Digestion:
Sleep:
Energy:
Focus:
Joint health:
Muscle strength:
Headaches:
Cycle regularity:
PMS:
Libido:
Food cravings:
Elimination regularity:

Food introduced:
Date:
Experience:

Food introduced:
Date:
Experience:

Food introduced:
Date:
Experience:

Food introduced:
Date:
Experience:

Food introduced:
Date:
Experience:

Food introduced:
Date:
Experience:

Thirty-Day Reintroduction Journal

Week 1

How I feel

_____
_____
_____
_____

Thoughts

_____
_____
_____
_____

My body

_____
_____
_____
_____

I AM focus

_____
_____
_____
_____

My stress strategy

_____
_____
_____
_____

My fitness

_____

_____

_____

_____

Journaling notes

_____

_____

_____

_____

_____

_____

_____

_____

_____

_____

_____

Thirty-Day Reintroduction Journal

Week 2

How I feel

_____
_____
_____
_____

Thoughts

_____
_____
_____
_____

My body

_____
_____
_____
_____

I AM focus

_____
_____
_____
_____

My stress strategy

_____
_____
_____
_____

My fitness

_____
_____
_____
_____

Journaling notes

_____
_____
_____
_____
_____
_____
_____
_____
_____
_____
_____

Thirty-Day Reintroduction Journal

Week 3

How I feel

_____

_____

_____

_____

Thoughts

_____

_____

_____

_____

My body

_____

_____

_____

_____

I AM focus

_____

_____

_____

_____

My stress strategy

_____

_____

_____

_____

My fitness

_____
_____
_____
_____

Journaling notes

_____
_____
_____
_____
_____
_____
_____
_____
_____
_____

Thirty-Day Reintroduction Journal

Week 4

How I feel

_____

_____

_____

_____

Thoughts

_____

_____

_____

_____

My body

_____

_____

_____

_____

I AM focus

_____

_____

_____

_____

My stress strategy

_____

_____

_____

_____

My fitness

_____

_____

_____

_____

Journaling notes

_____

_____

_____

_____

_____

_____

_____

_____

_____

_____

_____

CHAPTER 13

Buddha Belly Wrap-Up and Recipes

SO MUCH HAS manifested in the previous four years since the original publication of *Buddha Belly* in 2016. This book is now a foundational piece of the educational process for my school, the Holistic Wellness Coaching Academy, where we train and certify new and experienced coaches and professionals in gut health and mindset coaching. As of *Buddha Belly*'s rerelease, we have trained hundreds of coaches in over twelve different countries and counting! These passionate individuals are utilizing the concept of holistic gut health to impact the entire world and empower a new level of wellness and well-being based on nature's design. While you are encouraged to start your Buddha Belly journey with this book, for those who may need more assistance from a trained and certified coach or those considering becoming a certified coach, you can find all of that information at guthealthschool.com.

Along my own health journey and since the original release of *Buddha Belly* in 2016, I have been blessed to meet so many people who have contributed their own experience with gut health. Women have shared their experience using the Buddha Belly gut protocol to overcome infertility resulting in a healthy pregnancy. Men have shared their experiences using Buddha Belly to reset their hormones, lose weight, and sleep better. From migraine improvement to weight loss, thyroid balancing, anxiety, depression, and more, many people have shared how Buddha Belly and gut health have empowered their lives. I have been my own testimonial as well.

What I discovered along my journey while writing and living Buddha Belly was something more complex than just an improved physical state. Physically, I was able to return to my prebaby weight while breastfeeding, which is something that has always been very difficult for me. I also experienced less joint and muscle pains, improved digestion, loss of sugar addiction, and no seasonal allergies for the first time in ten years. These improvements were exciting and affirming, but the most powerful changes for me were in my mind. Becoming aware of my self-perception and motivating myself with a nurturing love has brought so much more peace into my life. Until this point, I had thought that a chronic state of stress was normal, and I never could have imagined ditching the little voice that would constantly break me down by relentlessly critiquing my physical body. I have not mastered these areas, and to be one hundred percent honest, I reread the chapters on stress and self-appreciation frequently, but I don't do this out of vanity. I read through these chapters when I feel myself forgetting to live the way I preach to others. It is much easier to show love or encourage another to love themselves than it is to love yourself. Doing this reminds me to show myself the love, grace, and patience that I desire for everyone else. I am grateful for all the experiences that have brought me right where I am today and feel blessed to be able to lead many others to a similar life. A life that is truly healthy.

Coach Britt

For more recipes, supplement, gut testing, and health inspiration and to follow me, visit buddhabellycoach.com.

Buddha Belly Recipes

Smoothy Love

Clean Green

1 c. cucumber
4 oz. purified water
2 handfuls spinach
½ small lemon (whole)
4 ice cubes

Start with the water and then add cucumber and lemon. Blend well. Next add spinach and blend again until pureed. Lastly, add ice cubes and blend to your desired consistency.

Chocolate Chia Superfood

6 oz. almond milk
1.5 c. chopped kale
1 small frozen banana
2 tbs. chia seeds
2 tbs. cocoa powder

Start by combining milk, kale, and chia seeds in blender. Blend until kale is broken down well. Next add remaining ingredients and blend to desired consistency

Tropicolada

¼ c. coconut water
4 oz. canned coconut milk
½ c. frozen pineapple chunks
¼ c. unsweetened, flaked coconut
1 tbs. vanilla extract
4 ice cubes

Combine all ingredients except ice cubes to a pureed consistency. Lastly. add ice cubes and blend well.

Protein Berry Bliss

6 oz. almond milk
1 large handful spinach
2 scoops grass-fed collagen protein
½ c. frozen organic mixed berries

Combine almond milk and spinach and blend to break down greens. Add remaining ingredients and blend well.

Spicy After Party

¼ c. purified water
¼ c. lime juice
1 red bell pepper
½ c. chopped celery
2 c. chopped romaine
1 tsp. cayenne
1 tsp. Himalayan sea salt
5 ice cubes

Combine water, lime juice, and romaine and blend well. Add all remaining ingredients except ice and blend. Add ice and blend to desired consistency

Zesty Italian

4 oz. clamato juice
2 Roma tomatoes
½ c. cucumber
1 tsp. Italian herbs
1 tbs. olive oil
1 tsp. black pepper
5 ice cubes

Blend all ingredients except ice until well pureed. Add ice and blend to desired consistency.

Very Huckleberry Healthy

6 oz. unsweetened almond milk
½ small avocado
1 c. chopped kale
½ c. frozen huckleberries

Combine first three ingredients and blend well. Add huckleberries and blend to desired consistency.

Tropi-kale Protein Smoothie

4 oz. unsweetened almond milk
4 oz. coconut water
½ small avocado
1.5 c. chopped kale
1 serving grass-fed collagen protein
1 c. frozen mango

Combine almond milk, coconut water, avocado, and kale and blend well. Add remaining ingredients and blend to desired consistency

Banana Nut Breakfast

8 oz. unsweetened almond milk
1 frozen banana
1 tbs. almond butter
1 tsp. cinnamon
1 tbs. Maple syrup
1 tsp. maple extract
3 ice cubes

Combine all ingredients except ice and blend well. Add recommended ice or enough to achieve desired consistency.

Pumpkin Protein Spice

4 oz. canned coconut milk
1 frozen banana
½ c. pureed pumpkin
1 tbs. almond butter
1 serving, grass-fed collagen protein powder

Combine all ingredients in a high-powered blender and blend to desired consistency.

Creamy Chocolate Omega

6 oz. unsweetened almond milk
½ small avocado
2 tbs. chia seeds
1.5 c. chopped spinach
½ frozen banana
2 tbs. cocoa powder
3 ice cubes

Combine the first four ingredients and blend well. Add remaining ingredients and blend to consistency.

Sweet Green Apples

6 oz. coconut water
1 small green apple
1 c. spinach
1 c. kale
½ small lemon (with rind)
5 ice cubes

Blend all ingredients except ice. Blend well to break down fiber. Add ice and blend to desired consistency.

Mango Macro Miracle

8 oz. coconut water

1 c. microgreens of choice (mint, parsley, etc.; experiment with
them all!)

2 tbs. chia seeds

½ c. frozen mango

Combine coconut water with greens and chia seeds and blend
well. Add frozen mango and blend to consistency.

RaspBelly-Biotic

6 oz. kefir (coconut milk kefir or raw goats milk kefir)
1 c. chopped kale
½ c. chopped leek
1 c. frozen organic raspberries
1 tbs. raw honey
1 tsp. vanilla extract

Combine kefir, kale, and leek and blend well. Add frozen berries and blend to desired consistency.

Full Belly Salads

Cajun Shrimp Superfood Salad

(Two large servings, four small servings)

3 large handfuls kale
1 c. quinoa (uncooked)
1 lb. large shrimp
1 large avocado chopped
½ c. diced sweet onion
2 cloves garlic chopped
4 stalks celery chopped
4 tbs. olive oil
2 tbs. lemon juice
2 tsp. cumin
1 tsp. cayenne pepper
sea salt to taste

Start by preparing the quinoa. I like to recommend using a small Crock-Pot. Mix a 1:2 ratio of quinoa to water and let cook on low for about 1.5 hours. You can make extra in a large crock to use for other recipes. Wash and dry kale and chop into small pieces. Chop avocado, garlic, and celery. Use half of the cumin and cayenne and sprinkle on shrimp. Combine olive oil and lemon juice with remaining spices including salt and set aside. Add all chopped ingredients along with shrimp and quinoa to a large bowl and toss with dressing mixture.

Blackberries and Turkey Salad with Blackberry Vinaigrette

(Two large servings, four small servings)

6 c. mixed greens
¾ c. chopped avocado
1 c. cooked turkey breast chopped
½ c. red onion thinly sliced
¼ c. slivered almonds
¾ c. c. blackberries whole

Blackberry vinaigrette

2 tbs, olive oil
2 tbs. white wine vinegar
1 tbs. raw honey
½ c. blackberries
1 tsp. sea salt

Chop all ingredients, toss together lightly, and set aside in a large bowl. Mix dressing in a blender, bullet, or food processor and puree well. Toss dressing into salad. You can choose to leave the almonds and whole blackberries out until the end allowing you to garnish them on top of the salad, making for a much more esthetically appealing plate.

Smoked Salmon Cobb with Coconut Ranch

(Two large servings or four small servings)

6 c. romaine chopped
1 c. cherry tomatoes sliced in half
½ red onion sliced into fine pieces
4 hardboiled eggs
6 oz. smoked salmon cut into bite-sized pieces
1 small avocado cut into chunks

Dressing

½ tsp. black pepper
½ tsp. chives
½ tsp. sea salt
¾ tsp. onion powder

¾ tsp. garlic powder
1 tbs. white wine vinegar
½ tsp. parsley
½ tsp. oregano
1 can of coconut milk (cream only)

Slice romaine, tomatoes, and onion and toss together. Slice hard-boiled eggs and add to the top of salad along with salmon and avocado. Mix dressing using some of the coconut liquid if necessary until you reach the desired consistency. Drizzle over entire salad or individual portions.

Pineapple Chicken Teriyaki Salad

6 c. chopped romaine
⅔ c. chunked pineapple (in 100% juice)
½ red onion sliced
1 orange bell pepper, sliced into strips
2 c. chicken breast cubed

Dressing

1.5 tbs. coconut aminos
2.5 tbs. extra virgin olive oil
2 tsp. honey
1 tbs. apple cider vinegar
½ clove garlic diced fine
⅛ tsp. ginger
sea salt to taste

Prepare chicken breast and set aside. Chop romaine, pepper, and onion and toss together in a large bowl. Add chicken and pineapple. In a separate container, mix dressing and pour over salad. Add salt to taste.

Protein-Packed Potato Salad

6 medium russet potatoes
½ purple onion diced
3 stalks celery chopped
3 hardboiled eggs
2 c. cubed chicken breast
1 large head romaine lettuce
4 tbs. olive oil
1 tbs. paprika
3 tsp. sea salt
2 tsp. black pepper
2 tbs. Italian seasoning
3 tbs. white wine vinegar
2 tbs. Worcestershire sauce
3 tbs. mustard

Wash and cook potatoes on a baking sheet at 375 for 50 minutes. Let cool completely and dice into chunks. Set aside. Chop onion, celery, eggs, chicken, and romaine and toss together in a large bowl. Drizzle potatoes with half the olive oil and all of the spices. Add spiced potatoes to bowl and toss. Combine remaining olive oil, mustard, vinegar, and Worcestershire sauce. Toss until coated evenly.

Sweet Chicken Dijon Salad

5 c. chopped romaine
1 c. chopped mustard greens
½ c. green onions
1 c. cooked quinoa
2 c. chicken breast cubed

Dressing

3 tbs. olive oil
2 tbs. Dijon mustard
2 tbs. raw honey
2 tbs. white wine vinegar
1 tsp. sea salt
2 tsp. black pepper

Mix dressing ingredients and set aside. Chop romaine, mustard greens, and onions and toss together. Add quinoa and chicken and mix well. Toss in dressing.

Nourishing Soups
and Sautés

Shrimp and Cauliflower Bone Broth Chowder

1 lb. cocktail shrimp
1 can full-fat coconut milk
16 oz. bone broth
1 tbs. coconut oil
1 medium head cauliflower
2 stocks celery
2 tsp. sea salt
1 tsp. black pepper
1 tbs. dill weed

In a large frying pan, heat coconut oil. Chop celery and cauliflower and add to the pan. Sauté the veggies until semifirm. Add remaining ingredients and cook on medium for another 5–10 minutes until heated through.

Mexican Chicken Chili

(Four medium portions)

1 lb. chicken breast sliced
1(14 oz.) can full-fat coconut milk
2 c. bone broth
1 can Mexican diced tomatoes (no sweetener)
1 (4 oz.) can diced green chilies
2 tbs. coconut oil
½ large sweet onion diced
4 stocks of celery diced
2 tbs. sea salt
1 tsp. chili powder
2 tsp. cumin

Chop chicken breast into medium strips and set aside. Dice onion and celery. In a large frying pan, heat coconut oil on medium heat. Dice onion and celery and add to the frying pan. Sauté veggies until semi softened. Add sea salt, chili powder, and cumin and cook for 1 minute. Pour coconut milk and bone broth over mixture and reduce heat slightly. Lastly, add cooked chicken and cook for another 4 minutes, stirring frequently

Egg Drop Quinoa Soup

(Two servings)

1 tbs. coconut oil
4 eggs
½ c. chopped chives
1.5 c. cooked quinoa
1.5 c. bone broth
½ c. water
2 tsp. basil
1 tsp. black pepper
sea salt to taste

Start by scrambling eggs in coconut oil and chopping into small pieces. Set aside. Next, heat bone broth on medium-low and add green onion. Heat for 5 minutes or until the desired temperature is reached. Be careful not to overheat, or you will lose the benefits of the bone broth. Add quinoa and egg along with seasoning. Add sea salt to taste.

This is a great soup to substitute instant noodles and processed chicken noodle.

Fajita Fri

(Two large servings, or four small servings)

1 red bell pepper
1 yellow bell pepper
1 medium yellow onion sliced into strips
2 c. broccoli straws
2 c. chopped chicken breast (cooked)
2 tbs. coconut oil
2 tbs. coconut aminos
1 tsp. cayenne pepper
1 tsp. chili powder
2 tsp. cumin
2 tsp. lime juice
sea salt

In a large frying pan or wok, add coconut oil and heat on medium. Chop onion and peppers and sauté lightly in coconut oil along with broccoli straws. Once the veggies are cooked to a semifirm consistency, turn the heat down to medium-low and add chopped chicken. Mix in remaining spices and toss to coat. Add sea salt to taste.

Sunny over Spinach

(Two large servings, or four small servings)

6 c. spinach
2 tbs. Coconut oil
1 tsp. sea salt
4 free-range eggs
Coconut aminos

In a large frying pan, add coconut oil and spinach. Sauté until lightly wilted but not fully cooked down. Add sea salt to the top of spinach and pat down to form a "nest" or semiflat surface. Crack eggs over top of spinach. Cover and cook on medium for approximately 3 minutes. Check eggs to determine your desired level of "done." Once the eggs are cooked to your liking, remove the pan from heat, let cool for 2 minutes, top with coconut aminos, and serve. The mixture should hold together in a frittata-like form.

Note: Meals like this are fast, simple, and healthy. You can prepare this for breakfast, lunch, or dinner and even add a side of cooked diced potatoes for those who need more calories.

Broccoli Steak Stir Fry

(Two large portions or four small portions)

5 c. whole organic broccoli
2 c. steak cubed
2 tbs. water
1 tbs. olive oil
2 tbs. Worcestershire
1.5 tbs. coconut aminos
1 tsp. black pepper
sea salt to taste

Start by cooking steak to the desired tenderness. Cut the steak into cubes before or after its cooked and set aside. Add water and broccoli to a large frying pan and cook, covered on medium heat, stirring occasionally. Cool broccoli until firm but not hard. Once done, turn the heat down to medium-low and stir in remaining ingredients. Cook for another 5 minutes.

Hearty Meals

Basil Balsamic Roasted Salmon over Herbed Quinoa

2 tbs. Worcestershire sauce
1 tbs. balsamic vinegar
1 tsp. basil
1 tsp. pink Himalayan sea salt
2 (4oz) wild salmon fillets

Herbed quinoa

2 c. cooked quinoa
1 tsp. basil
1 tsp. onion powder
1 tsp. rosemary
2 tsp. sea salt (or to taste)
1 tsp. black pepper
2 tbs. olive oil

Preheat the oven to 375. Mix the Worcestershire sauce and vinegar and pour over salmon fillets in a deep rimmed baking dish or pan. Sprinkle basil and salt over fillets and bake for 18 minutes or until done.

For the quinoa, heat oil over medium heat in a frying pan and add quinoa. Heat until slightly crisp. Add remaining ingredients and cook another 2 minutes.

Serve salmon over a bed of quinoa or on the side and next to a large helping of steamed veggies or salad.

Deep-Dish Pizza with Quinoa Crust

2 c. cooked quinoa
2 tbs. Italian seasoning
1 tbs. sea salt
2 fresh eggs
1 tbs. olive oil

Start by preheating the oven to 350. Mix all ingredients for the crust in a medium bowl. Grease a 10–12-in. pie pan with olive oil and press quinoa mixture down into it and against sides. Bake for 15 minutes or until golden brown.

Topping options

Pizza sauce (no sweetener added)
Avocado slices
Onions
Olives
Pesto sauce
Chicken
Smoked salmon
Mushrooms

The possibilities are endless as long as they are clean so get creative and indulge in a favorite food that is healthy for your belly.

Wild Tenderloin and Mushrooms

(Two large servings)

1 lb. of wild meat tenderloin (we use elk or venison)
2 lb. of sliced mushrooms of choice
2 tbs. grass-fed butter
1 whole white onion
2 tbs. Worcestershire sauce
Sea salt to taste

Chop mushrooms and onion into large pieces and set aside. In a large frying pan add 1 tbs. butter and tenderloin meat. Cook over medium heat until cooked through. Once done, remove meat and set aside. Sauté mushrooms and onions in leftover meat juice. Once cooked to a semisoft consistency, add in the meat and remaining ingredients. Heat together for another 3 minutes and serve.

BBQ Chicken-Stuffed Sweet Potatoes

(Four servings)

> 4 medium sweet potatoes
> ½ lb. organic free-range chicken breast diced
> ½ large white onion
> 1 tbs. olive oil
> 2 tbs. grass-fed butter
> sea salt to taste

BBQ sauce

> 6 oz. can of organic tomato paste
> 8 oz. organic applesauce
> 2 tbs. balsamic vinegar
> ¼ tsp. black pepper
> ½ tsp. onion powder
> ½ tsp. garlic powder
> ½ tsp. Worcestershire sauce
> ½ tsp. coconut aminos

Preheat oven to 400 degrees. Wash sweet potatoes and poke with knife three times. Cook potatoes at 400 degrees for 20 minutes and then turn the heat down to 350 for a remaining 60 minutes. Mix BBQ sauce ingredients and set aside. Cook diced chicken in a frying pan, and add 3 tablespoons of BBQ sauce. Cook for another 2 minutes and set aside. Chop onions and sauté in olive oil until softened. Add to chicken mixture. When potatoes are done, let cool slightly and cut slightly down the middle of each. Add butter and salt to potato and mash together. Top each potato with ¼ of chicken mixture.

Wild Shepherd's Pie

Filling

2 c. chopped mushrooms
1 can Mexican diced tomatoes
1 chopped onion
¾ c. olives diced
½ lb. ground meat (we used venison)
½ c. tomato paste
1 tbs. chili powder
1 tsp. cumin
½ tbs. salt

Topping

½ c. gluten-free flour
½ c. almond meal
1 tbs. honey
1 egg
½ c. almond milk
1 tbs. coconut oil
½ tsp salt

For the filling, start by chopping the onions and olives while cooking in a frying pan the ground meat of choice until thoroughly cooked. Next add all the remaining ingredients except for tomato paste until sautéed down a bit. Don't let veggies get too soggy seeing as how they will continue to cook in the oven, but this will help some of the moisture to leave the veggies. Next add tomato paste and seasonings and set aside.

Start your topping by mixing the gluten-free flour and almond meal along with salt. Next add the milk, honey, and coconut oil and set aside.

To combine I used two 4x8-in. loaf pans (double recipe for large family or leftovers) and split the filling between the two pans like pictured above. Next split the cornmeal topping between the two pans and spread over top. The filling won't be super thick, which allows this recipe to be less heavy than commonly prepared and very balanced with protein and veggies. (It's still so yummy!)

Bake in a preheated oven at 375 F for approx. 17 minutes. Once done, let cool for 5 mins and serve with a side salad or raw veggie of choice!

Smoked Salmon Quinoa Cakes

2.5 c. cooked quinoa
¾ lb. smoked salmon flaked or cut into small bits
4 eggs
½ c. onion diced
1 large clove garlic diced
2 tsp. sea salt
1 tsp. black pepper
2 tsp. dried basil
olive oil

Chop onion and garlic and set aside. In a large mixing bowl, beat all eggs well and add onion, garlic, salt, pepper, and basil and mix well. Fold in salmon and quinoa. Heat a nonstick pan to medium and coat with olive oil. Using ¼ measuring cup, scoop the mixture and place it in the pan. Flatten down into a ½-in. patty and cook each side until done (approx. 3 minutes each side). Serve with a large number of veggies or over a bed of greens.

Sweet Treats and Superfood Snacks

Frosted Fudgy Raw Brownies

2.5 c. pitted dates
¾ c. walnuts
½ c. cocoa powder
⅛ tsp. sea salt
1 tbs. coconut oil

Frosting

3 tbs. coconut oil
3 tbs. maple syrup
1 tsp. vanilla extract
½ c. cocoa powder

In a high-grade blender or food processor, add dates, walnuts, cocoa powder, salt, and coconut oil. Blend well until a crumbly but slightly sticky consistency results. In an 8x5 loaf pan, press the brownie mixture evenly and tightly. Mix frosting ingredients. If the oil is solid, you can melt it in a bowl by sitting the bowl in a pan of hot water.

Spread frosting mixture over brownies and place in the freezer for at least 15 minutes. Cut and serve. Brownies can be stored in a freezer, fridge, or room temp, but the frosting will change consistency depending on what temperature it is stored at.

You can experiment with the recipe by adding raspberry flavoring, mint, etc.

Macadamia Butter Bars

Bar ingredients

> 1 c. cashew butter
> ¼ c. coconut oil
> ¼ c. Maple syrup
> ¼ c. macadamia nuts
> ⅓ c. unsweetened coconut
> pinch of salt

White chocolate topping

> 1 tbs. coconut oil
> 2 tbs. Honey or maple
> ¼ c. coconut milk cream
> 1 tsp. vanilla
> ¼ c. unsweetened coconut

Start by melting the coconut oil and adding this and the cashew butter to a food processor along with maple and pulse for approx. 30 seconds and then add coconut and salt and pulse for another 20 seconds. Scrape mixture into a clean bowl and stir in Macadamia nuts. Line a loaf pan with parchment paper allowing it to hang over so it can be easily removed. (I used a 5x5 glass pan for thicker bars)

Pour the first part of the bar mixture into the pan and place it in the freezer.

Topping: Melt the coconut oil and add maple and vanilla; then fold it in the coconut cream. To get the coconut "cream," place a can of full-fat coconut milk in the fridge for a few hours, take the top off, and skim thick cream off the top. Use extra liquid in smoothies. Use the leftover liquid for smoothies or other healthy recipes."

Lastly, fold in ¼ c. coconut and pour over top of bars and place in the freezer for at least an hour or more.

Dark Chocolate Almond Bark

½ c. melted coconut oil
3 tbs. pure maple syrup
½ c. cocoa powder
½ c. raw almonds
1 tsp. pink Himalayan sea salt (optional)

Start by melting the coconut oil in a bowl set in a larger pan of hot water. Add syrup and cocoa powder and mix well. Add almonds and stir to coat.

Pour mixture into a 5x8 loaf pan and sprinkle sea salt on top. Place in the freezer for 30 minutes.

Break the bark into pieces and store in a container in the freezer.

Sweet Potato Fries

2 large sweet potatoes
2 tbs. olive oil
sea salt to taste

Preheat the oven to 375.

Wash and dry sweet potatoes and remove the skin. Chop into long fry slices or rounds approximately ¼ inch thick.

Coat the fries in olive oil and place a large baking sheet as separated as possible.

Sprinkle with sea salt and bake for 45 minutes.

At the 25-minute mark, remove fries and turn with a spatula to prevent uneven cooking.

Kale Chips

1 large bushel of kale
3 tbs. olive oil
sea salt to taste

Wash and dry kale really well. If need be, wash ahead of time and lay out to dry or use a paper towel.

Preheat the oven to 350.

Remove stem from kale and rip or tear into chip-size pieces.

Coat kale evenly in olive oil and spread over a large baking sheet.

Bake for 10 minutes and turn over with a spatula.

Cook for another 10 minutes or until crispy and slightly browned.

Kale chips make an easy and delicious side for any hearty meal as well as an excellent alternative to chips.

Teas

Electrolyte Tea

10 tsp. loose leaf tea (we recommend a fruity non-caffeinated variety)
½ gal. purified water
½ gal. mason jar
2 tsp. pink Himalayan sea salt
4 tbs. fresh lemon juice
4 tbs. raw honey (optional)

Brew tea by steeping loose leaves in hot water for at least 10 minutes before straining and let cool.

You can cold-brew it as well the night before by adding leaves to room temperature water and letting sit for 12–24 hours before straining.

Once the tea is brewed and warm but not hot, add remaining ingredients, mix until dissolved, and keep in a Mason jar in the fridge.

Coconut Spiced Chai

2 tsp. lose leaf spiced chai tea blend
16 oz. purified water

Heat the water until it's just about to boil.
Steep chai blend for at least 10 minutes for extra flavor.
While steeping, mix creamer.

Super coconut creamer

1 can organic coconut milk
12 oz. nut milk (unsweetened; I like almond)
2 tbs. melted down LOCAL, RAW HONEY
2 tsp. vanilla extract

You will firstly want to melt the honey down by putting it in a glass container and submerging the container in a bowl of very hot water for a few minutes (DON'T use a microwave! It kills off all those healthful bacteria and radiation, and it doesn't taste good.)

Next, add the remaining ingredients to a 20-ounce jar and mix well. Shake before each use to break up coconut particles.

Lemonade Kombucha

12 oz. kombucha (if making yourself, we recommend a combination of lemongrass and black tea)
1 tbs. honey
3 tbs. fresh lemon juice
4 oz. carbonated water

Warm the lemon juice slightly and dissolve honey into it.
Add to kombucha and mix well.
Top with carbonated water.

Increase recipe size for large quantities and keep in the fridge.

About the Author

a board-certified health and life coach and founder of the Holistic Wellness Coaching Academy, where she trains and certifies health coaches in gut health and mindset coaching. Brittney, popularly known as "Coach Britt," came to know the power of the microbiome after a lifetime of struggling with her own anxiety, depression, weight, and hormonal imbalances. By her early thirties, she had found an essential tool in defeating her constant challenges. This tool was the microbiome or better known as the human gut. After practicing as a board-certified health and life coach, she went on to teach gut health education to coaches and wrote the first addition to *Buddha Belly* in 2015.

Brittney has since enjoyed speaking, writing, educating, and leading coaches and wellness professionals. As the HWCA academy has grown, Brittney mainly focuses on training the coaches in what she refers to as "holistic gut health" and mentors them through utilizing their education to create and advance their wellness businesses and ventures. She has a strong passion for helping people cultivate life and defines a healthy life as a combination of mental, emotional, physical, and spiritual well-being. She believes that physical health is just a tool for living at our ultimate life's potential and that if we can motivate people toward purpose and fulfillment, then guiding them in self-care is easy because they are motivated for something far bigger.

Brittney was raised in the Pacific Northwest where she enjoys the incredible nature, a balance of leadership, and simplicity and still resides there today with her family.

CPSIA information can be obtained
at www.ICGtesting.com
Printed in the USA
LVHW071222120621
690023LV00001B/1